Why Even Good Doctors Make Mistakes

Why Even Good Doctors Make Mistakes

◆

An Anecdotal Introduction to Medicine

Jack Hasson, MD and Razi Sharafieh

iUniverse, Inc.
New York Lincoln Shanghai

Why Even Good Doctors Make Mistakes
An Anecdotal Introduction to Medicine

Copyright © 2005 by Jack Hasson and Razi Sharafieh

All rights reserved. No part of this book may be used or reproduced by any means, graphic, electronic, or mechanical, including photocopying, recording, taping or by any information storage retrieval system without the written permission of the publisher except in the case of brief quotations embodied in critical articles and reviews.

iUniverse books may be ordered through booksellers or by contacting:

iUniverse
2021 Pine Lake Road, Suite 100
Lincoln, NE 68512
www.iuniverse.com
1-800-Authors (1-800-288-4677)

ISBN-13: 978-0-595-34569-4 (pbk)
ISBN-13: 978-0-595-79316-7 (ebk)
ISBN-10: 0-595-34569-7 (pbk)
ISBN-10: 0-595-79316-9 (ebk)

Printed in the United States of America

Dedication: To medical students—past, present, and future

Contents

Preface xi

Part I: Introduction

Chapter 1 What Pathology Is and What Pathologists Do. 3
Chapter 2 The Background of These Anecdotes. 5

Part II: The Anecdotes

1951–52, Montefiore Hospital, New York, Internship . . . 11

Chapter 1 Welcome to Medicine 13
Chapter 2 The Devil Is in the Details. 16
Chapter 3 How to Prevent Acquiring Infectious Diseases from Patients. 20
Chapter 4 Exceptions Disprove Rules 23

1952–57, Montefiore Hospital, New York, Training in Pathology 27

Chapter 5 A Harmless Looking Lump 29
Chapter 6 How a Benign Tumor Can Kill. 32
Chapter 7 How Fast Can a Cancer Grow? 34
Chapter 8 Looks Aren't Everything 37

1957–66, The Jewish Hospital of St. Louis, Missouri, Director of Laboratories.... 41

CHAPTER 9	Managing an Insoluble Problem..............	43
CHAPTER 10	A Humiliating Mistake	46
CHAPTER 11	A Pathologist's Nightmare	50
CHAPTER 12	Wow! A New Disease!	58
CHAPTER 13	A Hopeless Case with a Happy Ending	63
CHAPTER 14	No Help from the Best and Brightest...........	66
CHAPTER 15	Two Deceptive Breast Tumors................	69
CHAPTER 16	A Deadly New Life Form....................	73

1966–73, Montefiore Hospital, New York City, Attending Pathologist 81

CHAPTER 17	The Mother of All Cancers...................	83
CHAPTER 18	A Stroke That Wasn't a Stroke................	86
CHAPTER 19	A Cancer Can Do Anything..................	88

1973–92, Mount Sinai Hospital, Hartford, Connecticut, Chief of Pathology..... 91

CHAPTER 20	A Rare Cause of a Rare Disease	93
CHAPTER 21	The Jogger Who Fainted	97
CHAPTER 22	An Unforgivable Sin........................	100
CHAPTER 23	A Delayed Bomb	103

1990–2000, The University of Connecticut Health Center, Farmington, Connecticut, Associate Professor of Pathology..... 107

CHAPTER 24	A Devastating Pregnancy	109

Chapter 25	Sudden Death	112
Chapter 26	The Doctors Never Heard of This One	116
Conclusion		121

Part III: Appendix

A. The Heart, Circulatory System, and Heart Failure 125

B. The Immune System 132

C. Studies on Diagnostic Errors 135

D. Two Common Diagnostic Errors.................. 136

E. A Comparison of Traditional and New Technological Diagnostic Methods................... 137

References.................................... 139

Acknowledgments............................... 141

Index... 143

Preface

Life expectancy in the United States was 62 years in 1935, when Congress passed the Social Security Act, which provided old age insurance. The latest available official life expectancy in 2001 was 77.2 years. At this rate, it is conceivable that life expectancy will exceed 78 years by the end of 2004. This progress is due to advances in medical knowledge and applied technologies, which often boggle the imagination. Hospitals, doctors, and health care plans confidently advertise their services implying customer satisfaction as expected with all services and products.

The bad news is a firestorm of medical litigation, which has been raging out of control for over thirty years and is still a crisis. This has caused medical costs to skyrocket and doctors to abandon medical practice or specialties prone to litigation. The most powerful tool of lifelong medical education for doctors has been the lessons learned from errors, the main theme of peer review conferences. The deliberate suppression of such educational conferences that might reveal litigious facts has crippled medical standards. The meetings concerning errors revealed at autopsy have also been suppressed and the autopsy is almost obsolete. Disharmony between patients and doctors has become a dark side of our culture. One wonders how much higher our life expectancy would be in the absence of these problems.

The causes of litigation are complex. Members of the state and federal legislatures usually fall into two opposing camps when considering remedial legislation. One blames greedy lawyers and the other blames greedy insurance companies. Neither one is the problem. They are each doing what they are supposed to do according to their rules. The more basic causes include a societal delusion that infallible medical care is possible and mandatory; a flawed jury system, which has led to bizarre astronomical settlements; and a flawed liability insurance structure, which provides funds for compensation of patient injury solely from the physicians' liability insurance.

These are monumental problems and there are no easy solutions. The purpose of these anecdotes is to illustrate how unpredictable medical practice can be in a small minority of cases and how this can lead to unavoidable errors. At the University of Connecticut Health Center, I frequently related entertaining anecdotes to my students to clarify an understanding of a disease with a case study having a dramatic happy or sad outcome. These anecdotes became popular because they stirred an emotional response matching my own as I related them and relived each as a happy memory or dismal nightmare. The students were unaccustomed to such emotional displays of real cases. My classes became popular because I brought the study of disease to life. My own physician on the faculty, Dr. Michael Grey, had heard of my entertaining style and suggested that I write up a collection of cases. I found great pleasure in recalling and writing them up because of all the associated wonderful memories. This collection is the result.

The suppression of educational conferences concerning medical errors—one of the dire consequences of rampant medical litigation—motivated me to write this book. Although one of the included cases was litigated, I emphasize that none of these anecdotes were intentionally selected as examples of medical litigation. The anecdotes only concern diagnostic problems often leading to wrong diagnoses. They illustrate why most diagnostic errors are unavoidable. Vast voids in knowledge cause errors as well as the endless variety of unexpected ways that Nature dictates how a disease will behave in a particular patient and mislead the doctor to the wrong diagnosis. My original intent was to publish these anecdotes for premedical and medical students to better prepare them to cope with these inherent uncertainties of medical practice. In medical school, the faculty repeatedly impressed us to study hard in order to accept the awesome responsibility for a human life. But the reality of uncertainty was never mentioned, as if it did not exist in the world of the well-informed physician. It took almost a lifetime for me to realize how insightful it would have been had I had been so prepared to cope with uncertainty upon entering medical school or even earlier. It then occurred to me that the average citizen might also benefit from an insight into medical practice that replaces its mystique with a clear idea of its capabilities and limitations. This may be at least a beginning to dispel the delusion of infallible medical practice.

Some knowledge about the details of how organs are structured and work and how diseases affect organs is necessary in order to follow some of the stories. The basic facts are not like rocket science but more like the rules of any sport. I have made liberal use of footnotes to elaborate on the meaning of unfamiliar technical words. I also prepared an illustrated explanation in the appendix of the structure and function of the circulatory system and heart, and a description of the immune system. These systems come up often enough in the anecdotes to give reason for one explanatory reference in the appendix concerning several anecdotes.

The anecdotes are presented in chronological sequence. They begin with my internship in 1951 at Montefiore Hospital in New York City followed by my career as a pathologist. They end in 2000 when I retired as an associate professor of pathology at the University of Connecticut Health Center in Farmington. I held five positions after my internship for variable periods. I experienced several of the anecdotes during each period. The anecdotes are arranged in the Table of Contents into five sequential groups with headings specifying the institutions, my titles and the duration of years in each one.

PART I

Introduction

1

What Pathology Is and What Pathologists Do

Pathology is the study of abnormal structural and functional changes in organs due to diseases and their causes. Giovanni Morgagni, a brilliant Italian physician and anatomist in the eighteenth century, initiated the first autopsy dissections leading to valid conclusions that stood the test of time. He sought what structural changes could be seen in organs injured by disease and how these changes accounted for symptoms.

Diseased organs usually can be easily recognized postmortem because they appear very different from normal organs, and the changes seen in a particular disease are major clues to its recognition. He described these changes in over 700 cases in a classic treatise in 1761. The technique of surgically dissecting organs postmortem to learn the structural basis for disease spread throughout Europe and culminated in a renaissance of medicine in Austria and Germany in the nineteenth and early twentieth centuries. Large medical centers developed in Vienna and Berlin, which included pathology institutes. The sole functions of these institutes were to perform autopsies, conduct research, and to teach pathology to both students and physicians.

Carl Rokitansky was a pioneer in the first half of the nineteenth century as head of the pathology institute in the Allgemeines Krankenhaus (General Hospital) in Vienna. He studied a total of thirty-thousand autopsies during his forty-year tenure or about 750 cases per year. This was a monumental achievement considering that the average yearly caseload for a medical examiner is 200 cases. His department became a center for postgraduate education of physicians from around the world, including many from the United States. In those days, the microscope was not yet in routine use, and it is incredible how much new knowledge he contributed with only naked-eye study of the organs on the operating table.

The next great leader in the second half of the nineteenth century was Rudolf Virchow, who headed the pathology institute in the Charity Hospital in Berlin, Germany. He revolutionized the postmortem examination by introducing the use of the microscope to study the cells in organs more closely. He led the way to most of the technology we still use today[1]. This was revolutionary because it sparked an explosion of new knowledge on structural changes due to disease by seeing the cellular changes associated with the changes obvious to the naked eye.

Pathologists, led by William Welch at Johns Hopkins University, who himself trained in the Austrian and German pathology institutes, set up departments of pathology in our medical centers in the early twentieth century. The techniques used to study the organs at autopsy quickly progressed to study the diseased tissues removed from living patients, giving rise to the subspecialty of surgical pathology. This field and its refinements became the dominant activity of pathologists in the ensuing years because of its immediate practical importance for the care of the living. Today, pathologists direct hospital diagnostic laboratories, which provide all of the laboratory tests including tissue biopsies that are essential to the diagnoses of diseases by physicians.

---

1. Virchow prepared very thin transparent slices of organs, measuring 2/10,000 of an inch thick. The slices are put on a thin glass slide, stained, and covered with a very thin, transparent piece of glass called a coverslip. These slices are stained with beautiful colorful dyes, which enable studying the details of individual cells microscopically.

2

The Background of These Anecdotes

When I was a medical student in the late 1940s, my fellow students and I were awed by the challenge of being responsible for a human life. The faculty reminded us of this in every phase of our education. Everything we learned was relevant. We dared not miss lectures or neglect our studies, which, we were led to believe, might later cost the life of a patient. Students eagerly attended medical conferences such as the weekly grand rounds, which concerned current patients with problems in diagnosis or treatment. They heard differences of opinion expressed among their role models, occasionally in the form of heated exchanges. The voids in contemporary medical knowledge and acknowledgment of nature's whimsical ways were heard loud and clear. We students became imbued with the imperative to keep abreast of new knowledge and to always be circumspect about every diagnosis so as to avoid errors.

One major conference attended by all was the clinico-pathologic conference or CPC. This was by far the most popular weekly conference. The chief pathologist selected an autopsied case that reflected a diagnostic problem during the decedent's life. A discussant, who did not know the actual diagnosis, presented a detailed review of the patient's illness, followed by an analysis of the possible diagnoses and concluded with a final diagnosis. The pathologist then presented the actual autopsy findings. Whether or not the discussant made the correct diagnosis mattered far less than the quality of the analysis. The discussion that followed the analysis and findings was the climax of the CPC. The role models in the audience engaged in exciting debates about diagnosis and therapy. The auditorium was always packed with enthusiastic doctors and medical students. The hour always seemed to end much too soon. Doctors conscientiously attended all of these conferences for the rest of their lives, regarding them as critical, intellectual exercises essential to maintaining their fitness to practice medicine.

The doctors of the pre-1970 era were, in a sense, applied scientists because they applied the scientific method, the basis for all new knowledge in the sciences, to their daily practice. The method requires that the acceptance of a new fact or theory must be supported by solid evidence and stand up to repeated tests. Doctors sharply defined the difference between proven diagnoses and diagnoses of diseases of unknown cause, where solid proof is often elusive or impossible to obtain. Their pursuit of autopsies was another example of the application of the scientific method, because autopsies were done as a last resort in order to finally establish the actual diagnoses in problematic patients. A firestorm of medical litigation began in the 1970s and has since led to radical changes in both medical practice and education. The number of lawsuits during that time reached 76 times the number occurring in the 1950s. The firestorm is still burning out of control. Jury awards exceed millions of dollars and skyrocketing premiums for medical liability insurance may even exceed physicians' incomes. Doctors have been forced to end practices in specialties prone to litigation such as obstetrics, or to relocate their practices to areas with lower insurance premiums as compared to states like Texas, Nevada, and Pennsylvania where such costs are greatest. The current liability insurance crisis is the worst one yet since its inception twenty years ago. Its effects on medical education and practice have been devastating.

Since the 1970s, many doctors, as well as the public, have acquired the mindset that medical practice must be flawless. For doctors, this point of view has meant that just one mistake could lead to litigation and threaten their careers. Ironically, the remarkable advances in medical knowledge and technology, which have enhanced diagnostic accuracy and treatments, have served to inflate the delusion of medical infallibility. Some practicing physicians who are also on the faculties of medical schools have conveyed the impression that perfection is an attainable goal and that all errors can be avoided. From this perception, many students no longer are filled with awe in anticipation of their future responsibilities. Instead they are filled with misguided confidence. They come to believe that they are destined to enter a profession where improved technology will continually eliminate any chance of error and guarantee that they will always "do good."

Advances in medical technology actually do not make all diagnoses foolproof, but do make more diseases subject to proven diagnoses. Many doctors still presume flawless practice and regard as routine accurate diagnoses based on laboratory and imaging technologies. Their gratifying successes with the great majority of their patients reinforce their hopeful presumption of infallibility. The doctor's approach to a patient has become more like the approach of a confident automobile mechanic to an engine than that of a cautious scientist striving to avoid diagnostic errors. If trends in medical education continue as they have in recent years, new doctors will be increasingly unprepared to both anticipate and cope with error. If students perceive their teachers as infallible divinities rather than as cautious, thoughtful scientists, they will embark on their careers with an inappropriate sense of confidence and empowerment.

Since the 1970s, doctors have inevitably made mistakes for which they were unprepared. Because they have been led to expect perfection, their first error inevitably engenders devastation. They often no longer discuss their errors at designated conferences with their peers, all of whom have also committed errors. Instead, because "flawless practice" is the current standard, the current trend is to conceal all errors and avoid any discussions about them. The possibility of medical litigation also encourages cover-ups. Revelations about an error at a peer review conference are subject to discovery in court. Admittedly, there are state laws that protect the content of peer review conferences from discovery in court in order to maintain their value for educating physicians. Nevertheless, loopholes have weakened these laws, thereby strengthening the aversion to peer review conferences.

The great tragedy of our time is that more and more doctors today share the delusion that they must be infallible. Tragically, many actually have no idea of their plight. They acquired the delusion from the first day of medical school and they accept their mind-set as the norm. Unlike their predecessors, these doctors are no longer "applied clinical scientists" because they have been brought up in an environment where the scientific method was abandoned. This is the legacy left to current medical practice by suppression of errors and the obsolescence of the autopsy. Today, doctors simply do not request autopsies in order to avoid litigation based on unexpected findings. Requesting an autopsy has become a first step in self-incrimination.

The following anecdotes will show that, in spite of spectacular medical advances, fixing a medical problem is not quite like the repair of an appliance or automobile. The automobile mechanic has a manual, which accounts for each part of the specific car model and year, down to the individual screws. Doctors also have "manuals" but they are nowhere near as complete. For example, more than half of the pages in an average textbook of medicine are devoted to diseases of unknown cause. This gives some idea of the vast holes in contemporary medical knowledge with which doctors must cope. Compared to an auto mechanic, the doctor is at a great disadvantage because each patient is vastly different from every other one. They cannot be categorized like a certain make or model of an automobile. However, we can loosely compare an individual patient to a custom built, one-of-a-kind car. The approach to such a machine would demand creative thinking by the mechanic obliged to attempt repairs by trial and error. Indeed, every human being is as unique as every other natural entity, like a mountain range, a hurricane, a lake, or a snowflake. Similarly, a disease in any individual human being is simply another unique natural phenomenon. Considering this uniqueness, doctors do extremely well by their patients. Moreover, given the ongoing increases in life expectancy and the advances in diagnostic and therapeutic progress that medical science has achieved over time, there is every reason to believe that most patients will benefit from this progress as the future unfolds.

Still, medical fallibility is unavoidable because the only way to end it is to end medical practice. This fallibility is due partly to the vast voids in medical knowledge, which make it virtually impossible for all diagnoses to be certain. Nature also generates fallibility by having diseases behave in unexpected ways and in guises that mimic one another. Admittedly, doctors do indeed make errors due to negligence, lack of knowledge, or bad judgment. These are examples of malpractice. However, they also make errors that are simply unavoidable and may or may not lead to patient injury. My hope is that both the public and doctors develop a more realistic expectation of high standards of practice that omits the delusion that there is such a thing as "flawless" medical care. "Flawless" practice should always be the goal of every doctor, but, realistically speaking, it is an unreachable star.

PART II

The Anecdotes

1951–52, Montefiore Hospital, New York, Internship

1

Welcome to Medicine

In the year 1951, when I was an intern in Montefiore Hospital, an 18-year-old Puerto Rican man was admitted because of advanced kidney disease. He was doomed to die because the failure of the kidneys to produce urine causes the retention of deadly wastes in the blood. The artificial kidney[1] was not yet invented and the only way to prolong life in those days was to carefully manage the intake of food and fluids with diet supplements. He was receiving the best possible care under the direction of the Chief of Medicine, Dr. Louis Leiter, who was a leading authority on kidney diseases. Dr. Leiter's interest in this subject was due to his near death from kidney disease himself as a boy.

It is important to note that Montefiore Hospital was known for its excellence at caring for chronic and often deadly diseases, with hospital stays for months and even years. This challenge attracted qualified residents in internal medicine like a magnet to learn the finest points of management of chronic lethal diseases. The great challenge was the identification and treatment of new symptoms, which could be due to the existing disease or to an entirely new treatable disease. This principle was gospel because of the natural tendency of a doctor to mistakenly attribute a new symptom to the existing incurable chronic disease.

This lad had moved to New York City ten years earlier to live with relatives, because his mother in Puerto Rico was too ill to care for him. Upon examining the patient, I was surprised to find clusters of raised scars, called keloids, deforming both of his elbows. This sort of scarring is often seen in healed third degree

---

1. An artificial kidney was developed in the early 1960s, which could maintain the lives of patients with kidney failure indefinitely by renal dialysis. It is a bedside mechanical device that circulates the patient's blood through it and filters out noxious chemicals, which are normally removed by a healthy kidney and eliminated as urine. Two tubes connect the patient's circulatory system to the mechanical system in the device. One tube carries the patient's blood to the device for cleansing and a second tube returns cleansed blood to the patient.

burns. I immediately realized that these scars had nothing to do with his kidney disease. He related that he repeatedly burned himself by leaning on hot room radiators with his elbows. These radiators were cast iron coils of pipe conducting steam heat and stood about three feet high, two feet long and less than a foot deep, and were a standard source of heat in apartments in New York City. The problem was that he had lost the sensations of pain and temperature in his elbows. That is why he burned himself repeatedly and never felt it.

This startling finding reminded me of a scene from a Hollywood movie I saw when I was eight or nine years old, which gave me nightmares. The setting was a tropical scene with two Americans in white suits, sitting opposite each other on a train going through a jungle. One of the two men was smoking a cigarette, which he held between his index and middle fingers. The other was shocked to realize that his smoking companion was unaware that his cigarette had burned down to his skin without any pain reaction. As the story unfolded, it turned out that leprosy was the cause of the loss of sensation in his fingers. This terrified me because of discussions about leprosy between my parents, which revealed that it was the worst of all diseases because it could destroy the face including the eyes, nose, mouth, and ears.

My memory of this movie prompted me to test his awareness of pinpricks, and I mapped out matching areas of complete anesthesia in both arms around the elbows. My basic medical education indicated that there were two possible causes for this disability. One was a local lesion in the center of the spinal cord such as a tumor, which destroyed the nerve tracts that transmitted pain and temperature skin sensation to the brain from both matching sides of the body. The other was actual destruction of the matching nerves in both arms by leprosy. I recorded these possibilities in the chart, but the resident physician, who was my supervisor, disagreed with my findings. His examination revealed that the patient did feel pain, when excessive force was applied to the scarred areas. Consequently, he overlooked the possibility of loss of sensation confined to the skin, dismissing leprosy as a possible cause.

Six months later, the patient developed early hints of the facial deformities of leprosy in the form of focal thickening of the skin on the forehead, which alerted the medical staff to the possibility of leprosy. A skin biopsy was diagnostic of leprosy. The commotion began when it was realized that a lowly intern had already considered the diagnosis on admission. For awhile, interns and residents were jokingly referring to leprosy as "Hasson's Disease," instead of its true medical name, which is "Hansen's Disease" after the discoverer of the causative germ. I basked in the admiration of my peers rather than reveal the secret of my diagnostic triumph.

Later on the staff spoke to his relatives and learned that his mother's disabling disease was leprosy, which led to his coming to live with them. Leprosy is extremely rare in the United States and the cases diagnosed each year are usually contracted in the tropics before settling here. It took ten years for the disease to appear, which is characteristic of the occasional long incubation periods in leprosy.

2

The Devil Is in the Details

The year was 1951 during my internship at Montefiore Hospital in New York. I admitted an 86-year-old man who appeared shrunken from weight loss, due to a loss of appetite for several weeks. I had no idea then whether he was aware that his referring doctor suspected the presence of a silent cancer that had spread to other organs without causing symptoms. Loss of appetite and profound weight loss over several weeks is an indication of many different diseases including cancer of any type, chronic infection, diseases of the immune system, and other rare diseases.

The patient was intelligent and seemed resigned to the fact that Montefiore Hospital was a place where many patients ultimately died and that he was a typical example. He was very cooperative, as if he was wondering whether he might be one of the lucky patients who would survive. I took a painstaking history of his illness, which only confirmed the findings of his referring doctor, without any new details that would suggest other diagnoses. In short, he seemed to be in good health in spite of his rapid decline. I reviewed the case with my supervising assistant resident, who had nothing to add. We then reviewed the case with our attending physician, who would be responsible for the management of this patient and whose decisions were final. We all agreed that the best course was to do all we could to see if a silent cancer could be demonstrated. This would possibly benefit the patient if our search revealed a hidden infection that we could treat and cure. Blood chemical studies were done to see if there were any diagnostic changes indicating spread of a cancer to skeletal bone. Samples of stools and urine were taken for evidence of hidden bleeding. A routine batch of X-rays was taken of the skeleton to see if there was any evidence of spread of a cancer to bone. A chest X-ray was taken to see if there were any shadows suggesting a lung cancer or spread of any cancer to both lungs. The negative results of all these studies were frustrating.

Hoping to save his life, we decided that we had to search more aggressively for a silent cancer with three more X-ray studies, involving enemas administered prior to the procedures and the physical discomfort of getting X-rays with an enema in place. He underwent an X-ray study of the kidneys first, which involved having a prior enema and then an intravenous injection of a radio-opaque dye. The dye outlined the details of kidney structures as it was carried by blood passing through the kidneys and was eliminated into the urine. The kidneys were normal. Another cleansing enema was followed by an enema of radio-opaque barium to visualize the large intestine on X-rays. This revealed no tumors or evidence of infection in the wall of the colon. The final study was an upper GI (gastrointestinal) series. The patient had to drink a barium solution, which flowed down the esophagus and into the stomach, making all these structures more visible on X-rays. Again, the studies were negative. In addition, his blood studies showed no hint of infection or an immune disease.

We were stumped, as sometimes happens in baffling cases, and had no choice but to give up and send the patient home with the support of a nutritious diet and multivitamins. The assistant resident reviewed the details in the patient's record before initiating his discharge from the hospital and told me that there was no record of two routine studies that were frequently done. These were a venous pressure and circulation time. The intern usually did these procedures as screening tests for heart failure when there was any suspicion of heart failure[1]. This would be considered if there was unexplained shortness of breath, or swelling of the ankles with a progressive increase in weight due to water retention, or unusual weakness in performing activities of daily living. For the sake of completeness, he asked me to do these tests before he could sign the discharge order. I agreed, but somewhat begrudgingly. Assistant residents often ordered interns to do procedures that they would not do themselves if an intern were not around.

The venous pressure was obtained by sticking a vein in the arm of the reclining patient with a needle that is connected to a pressure gauge. This is a measure of the blood pressure of venous blood returning to the heart and is normally one tenth of the usual arterial pressure. The higher arterial pressure results from the forceful contraction of the heartbeats propelling blood out of the heart and to the entire body. His venous pressure was normal. An elevated venous pressure would have suggested heart failure, among other possibilities but a normal venous pressure did not rule out heart failure. The final answer was given by the circulation time, which measured how fast blood is moving through the circulatory system. The time it takes for blood to go from one place to another is usually slowed down in heart failure. We used the following test to get this information. A

---

1. See Appendix A.

chemical was injected into a vein in the arm and a stopwatch would be started as soon as the injection was completed. The chemical caused a sudden extremely bitter taste in the mouth when it reached the tongue and caused the patient to suddenly grimace involuntarily and alert the intern to click the stopwatch off. The upper limit of a normal circulation time under these conditions was 16 seconds. This is the time it would take for blood to flow from the vein in the arm back to the heart and then into the lungs to pick up oxygen and then back to the heart to be ejected to all organs including the sensitive tongue. I was amazed to find that his circulation time was almost 40 seconds, which was grossly abnormal and indicated heart failure.

This was baffling because he lacked the usual symptoms or findings on physical examination. He looked worse now than he did on admission after all the physical stress we caused by the debilitating tests, which aggravated his loss of appetite. The assistant resident contacted our attending physician and I was instructed to initiate digitalis treatment for heart failure at once. Digitalis was the drug of choice in those days because of its remarkable though not understood beneficial effect on the failing heart. It had already been in use for heart failure for over a century. I ordered the drug with enthusiasm with the hope that we were on the right tract. One of the most gratifying experiences of my life was to visit him one morning a few days later when I encountered a beaming patient out of bed behaving with the vigor of someone about twenty years younger. He had already had a hearty breakfast and was clean-shaven after a shower. He asked me what it was that he was getting that made him feel reborn, and I explained the treatment to the best of my ability. I was embarrassed by the reverential manner in which he regarded me. He was soon discharged and followed in our cardiology clinic. What did all this mean? The answers came within a few days of digging into the books and presenting the case at Grand Rounds, our major weekly conference. There were two big unanswered questions. First, what was the nature of this mysterious heart disease with no usual symptoms and physical signs? The immediate answer was that we did not know. There is a type of heart disease called a "cardiomyopathy," which is an impressive tongue twister that simply means that something is wrong (pathy) with the heart (cardio) muscle (myo), but we do not know what it is. This is still a useful wastebasket term to categorize such cases. There are actually several different kinds of cases that fall into this category of heart disease. They are revealed at autopsy and may be impossible to distinguish during life. It must be added that even the autopsy sometimes fails to identify the kind of obscure disease that can silently eventually cause heart failure.

The other question is the explanation for the way this patient presented with loss of appetite and weight with associated weakness and nothing more. We did find reference to cases that have these symptoms due to heart failure. Apparently, the slowing of the circulation in these unusual cases targets the intestines by impairing the ability to absorb nutrients into the bloodstream from the intestinal contents causing a wasting of the body due to malnutrition. Somehow, this also causes a complete loss of appetite. Indeed, this has been called the "cachexia (wasting away) of heart failure."

This case occurred in 1951 and diagnostic procedures and treatments have changed ever since. The venous pressure and circulation times are no longer done. The technology of cardiac catheterization, which consists of threading delicate long tubes through veins into various chambers of the heart, has replaced the old methods. The new methods provide more information with greater accuracy. The circulation time was discontinued after a few short years of use because some patients died suddenly from an allergic reaction to the injected chemical agent. Today an imaging study using ultrasound, which visualizes the beating heart accurately, determines the presence of heart failure.

As for the treatment of heart failure, it is clear that the newer drugs in use today are even more effective than digitalis, which is still used by cardiologists for specific indications. It is no exaggeration to say that lives have been prolonged for years in patients with heart failure by drugs called ACE-inhibitors, beta-blockers, and aldactones. These drugs were originally used to treat hypertension, but a happy unexpected side effect was a remarkable effectiveness in heart failure of any cause as well. But it should come as no surprise to the reader that how these drugs work is unknown and the subject of intensive research.

3

How to Prevent Acquiring Infectious Diseases from Patients

I had just begun a six-week assignment on the tuberculosis service, consisting of two hundred men and women. These beds were located on the second and third floors of the south wing, a block-long three-story building with the women in the west wing and the men in the east wing. The assistant resident greeted me and briefed me on the special needs of these patients. He was anxious about precautions I must take to avoid getting infected. He told me to wear a mask whenever I contacted patients and showed me where I could always find one. His manner implied that this was one of the rules of the service.

The first patient I admitted was a young married woman in her early twenties who had recently given birth to her first baby a few months before admission. She was weeping quietly when I walked into her room and the weeping continued unchanged thereafter, which I realized meant a deep sorrow unrelieved by the distraction of my arrival. After I was satisfied that she saw my face and knew what I looked like, I put on the mask with great misgivings. I couldn't help but feel that I had intensified her sorrow as an outcast of society.

We exchanged a few words interrupted by sobs, and I was struck for the first time by the real depth of her sorrow when she told me that she had learned that she would be hospitalized for up to two years. After physicians decided the extent of the disease and its treatment, she was destined to spend most of that time at Montefiore Hospital's Bedford Sanitarium in Bedford Hills, Westchester County. She was devastated by the prospect of being separated from her first baby for all that time. Guilt overwhelmed me for wearing the mask and prompted me to remove it, regardless of my superior's warning. I subsequently learned from her that she had no symptoms and that the disease was discovered on a chest X-ray, which revealed a telltale shadow. A sputum test for tuberculosis was positive. In hindsight, I do believe that my taking off the mask had a positive effect. The chief of the service, Dr. Robert Bloch, who was nationally known, justified my bold action later.

He visited each patient on regularly scheduled patient rounds every Friday morning. I looked forward to his rounds and was promptly there before he arrived. The assistant resident showed up with a mask, wary of the many exposures to infection as we went from patient to patient. I wore no mask because there was no point in doing so now that I was already repeatedly exposed, and regarded the mask inimical to patient relations. Dr. Bloch appeared with his associate, Dr. Abraham Buchberg, and I immediately noticed that they wore no masks. I was pleasantly surprised and the assistant resident was obviously upset. I recall an exchange of words between him and Dr. Bloch, which went something as follows: Resident: "Why don't you wear a mask?" Dr. Bloch: "Because it doesn't do any good." Resident: "Does that mean I can still get infected?" Dr. Bloch: "Yes." Resident: "Then what can I do to prevent infection?" Dr. Bloch: "Get out of medicine." Dr. Bloch was a great teacher and a very warm human being, but he had no patience with impossible goals.

I had never really considered the risk of acquiring an infection from a patient until this experience. Many of the new cases of tuberculosis prove to have acquired the infection from someone in their environment with active disease. Physicians are similarly at risk. Indeed, one of my patients was a young internist getting treated, and I have personally known one other internist and two pathologists with cured infections. This is one of the dangers that make medical practice an adventurous profession.

Practically all of the cases were infectious because they fell into one of three groups. There were the recent admissions of new patients, who were infectious because of a positive sputum examination for the tubercle bacillus, which is diagnostic of the disease. These new cases were eventually transferred to the Bedford Sanitarium after physicians determined the extent of disease and decided a program of long-term anti-tubercular treatment. The patients stayed in the sanitarium anywhere from many months to a few years to encourage healing of lung infections by bed rest. The progress of these cases was followed with monthly X-rays and periodic sputum studies for live tubercle bacilli.

The second group consisted of active patients with special problems getting anti-tubercular and other treatments for infections of the lungs and also other organs. Some of these cases were transferred back to Montefiore Hospital from the sanitarium. They were readmitted to undergo surgical excision of unresponsive infections that resisted natural healing and were a continuing source of smoldering infection.

The third group consisted mostly of patients who were almost hopeless. The variety of cases that comprised this group reflected the spectrum of different forms of tuberculosis, which depended on the variable natural resistance of patients to infections. Those with the least resistance were subject to rampant infections such as tuberculous pneumonia, which was often fatal. Those with good resistance with far advanced old lesions were subject to a deadly disease that can occur in any long-standing chronic infection called amyloidosis[1].

Another type of hopeless case was a young woman with manageable tuberculosis, but who also had a slow growing malignant brain tumor that was impossible to remove surgically. It is worth noting that in those days there was also a huge number of undetected cases of tuberculosis in New York City, comprising more than 90% of the population. The immune systems of these people made them resistant to tuberculosis. They overcame their silent infections. They were not infectious to others because their sputums were free of tubercle bacilli. They were detected by a positive skin test for tuberculosis, which remained positive for years after the initial infection. The reason for the high rate of infection in New York City was the crowding. It was said that daily use of the New York City subways assured the unwary passenger of an eventual positive skin test.

---

1. The term "amyloid" refers to an abnormal protein, which permeates the organs and accumulates to the extent of interfering with their functions. Imagine how the network of thin cement between bricks in a brick wall would look if it tripled in thickness and shoved the bricks further apart. This is how amyloid infiltrates organs between cells and mechanically disrupts whatever the organ does. The amount of this protein, which is easily seen under the microscope, can double the weight of an organ and be fatal when the liver, heart, or kidneys are involved. Much has been learned about amyloidosis in the past fifty years, but how it is actually triggered and treated is unknown. There appears to be some relationship between the development of amyloidosis and the immune system (See Appendix B).

4

Exceptions Disprove Rules

During my internship on the cancer service in 1952, I admitted a stoical gentleman in his seventies who was resigned to dying from a cancer of the immune system called multiple myeloma[1], the cancer of plasma cells. A small number of plasma cells is normally found in the bone marrow. The referring doctor based the diagnosis on characteristic blood chemical changes and X-rays of bones, which showed multiple discrete round defects in bone structure due to the destructive tumor. The patient was debilitated with weight loss and anemia, which was obvious from the pale fingernails lacking shades of pink. The diagnosis had not yet been proven by a biopsy of the bone marrow.

The physical examination supported the original diagnosis. The laboratory report indicated an elevated concentration of calcium in the blood associated with a low phosphorous. This is characteristic of multiple myeloma and is due to bone destruction, which results in the breakdown of calcium compounds that give bone its rock hard consistency. The compounds dissolve into the bloodstream thereby raising the calcium concentration.

Being highly motivated and skeptical about accepting an unproven diagnosis of cancer, I eagerly considered other causes of the same blood calcium changes with bone destruction, especially a curable cause. A benign tumor of a parathyroid gland[2] can cause the same findings and can be removed surgically. I wishfully entered into the record a diagnosis of benign parathyroid tumor causing the disease called hyperparathyroidism as my first diagnosis with multiple myeloma as a second choice.

The patient died unexpectedly the day after admission before any diagnostic studies were done. The family agreed to an autopsy. I was keenly interested in the

---

1. The term myeloma is derived from the Greek *myelos*, which means bone and the suffix *oma*, which means tumor. The disease is called multiple myeloma because it usually appears as numerous tumors throughout the skeleton. This is a cancer of plasma cells, one of the types of cells that form the immune system (See Appendix B).

findings and visited the autopsy operating room. The pathologist was not yet finished, but had exposed the vertebra, the bones of the backbone. With a saw, the pathologist shaved a slice of bone off the surface of the backbone to expose the bone marrow cavity within. Normal bone marrow looks like a bright red sponge, but feels like a porous rock because of the network of the supporting bony framework. The vertebral bone in this case did have a normal appearance and bony consistency in most places, but also revealed soft round red-brown areas lacking bone. The pathologist diagnosed it as multiple myeloma. I asked her if the changes due to hyperparathyroidism could look like this. She did not know and suggested getting a quick answer by my looking at a smear of the bone marrow under the microscope. Normally, plasma cells make up only 1% or less of the many cell types that compose bone marrow. The smear revealed only malignant looking plasma cells and no normal marrow cell types, proving a diagnosis of multiple myeloma. I was disappointed but took comfort in the fact that my diagnostic analysis followed the rules.

A few weeks later, the resident pathologist who performed the autopsy greeted me and called me a genius. She explained that her microscopic study of the parathyroid glands showed no single tumor as expected, but did show microscopic changes in all four glands diagnostic of a rare cause of hyperparathyroidism called diffuse hyperplasia. Normal glands contain fatty tissue. All the fatty tissue is replaced in this disease by a proliferation or hyperplasia of enlarged benign parathyroid cells.

Obviously, I was no genius but just lucky. One of the guiding rules in diagnosing any disease is to explain all the clues in one patient with no more than one diagnosis. Mother Nature is not so obliging and contributes to our uncertainty by presenting cases with two and sometimes (but rarely) more major diseases. This is especially true in the aged. It happens that the dominant symptoms of one major disease may mask those of another that is missed and untreated. The failure of the doctors to identify the hyperparathyroidism in this case was unavoidable because of its rarity and having the same chemical findings as multiple

---

2. There are four parathyroid glands, a pair on each side of the back of the larger thyroid gland in the lower neck. Each is about double the size of a lentil bean and colored tan. These glands secrete a protein into the blood, a hormone, which maintains the blood calcium within a normal concentration range. The hormone's action is for the bone to release its calcium compounds into the blood should the calcium concentration fall. Normal calcium levels suppress the secretion of hormone. A benign tumor of one or more glands is not suppressed by increasing calcium levels and can secrete uncontrolled amounts of hormone that can melt away skeletal bone.

myeloma. The oversight made no difference in the fatal outcome due to multiple myeloma. If the same initial symptoms, signs and laboratory studies were, indeed, due to a parathyroid tumor rather than multiple myeloma, the microscopic study of the bone marrow would have revealed a normal picture without a hint of malignant plasma cells. Today, the diagnosis of hyperparathyroidism is easily confirmed preoperatively by measuring the concentration of the parathyroid hormone in the blood, which would be abnormally elevated.

1952–57, Montefiore Hospital, New York, Training in Pathology

5

A Harmless Looking Lump

During my first year residency in pathology in 1952, I was called to the operating room one day to be present for the excision of a chest wall tumor in a young man in his thirties. The patient was already anesthetized when I arrived and was lying on his left side with the right side of his chest facing upwards. His body was covered with sterile sheets except for the head and a rectangular 12- by 8-inch window exposing the skin of the right side of the chest. The skin was painted with iodine and framed by neatly placed surgical towels secured together with towel clips in the corners. The surgeon looked up and pointed out a bulge in the chest wall indicating an underlying tumor about 3 inches long and 2 inches wide. The mass was barely mobile by sideways pressure because of the confining overlying skin, which was stretched tight. We briefly exchanged comments on the nature of the tumor, which we realized was a tumor of the soft tissues in the chest wall overlying the rib cage. The soft tissues include muscle, fat, blood vessels, and nerves and each one can give rise to both benign and malignant tumors. This was my first experience with a soft tissue tumor, which are uncommon. The average general surgeon might see only one case per year.

The surgeon made a single neat 4-inch lengthwise cut through the skin along the middle of the bulge. A tan-yellow tumor literally popped out and came to rest loosely attached to underlying tissues framed by the relaxed loose flaps of skin. The surgeon seemed pleased that he did not have to do any fine dissecting since he peeled it off its bed so easily by just using his fingers. He placed the mass in a sterile tray and gave it to the circulating nurse who then gave it to me. He was obviously proud of such a rapid, neat operation. I had no idea what variety this soft tissue neoplasm was and the surgeon expressed no opinion. The surgeon proceeded to sew the loose skin flaps together to cover the raw bed of the tumor, and I brought the tumor to the surgical pathology laboratory.

The tumor was firm but compressible and had a slightly irregular surface. This tumor had no capsule, which is an enclosing shell with a very smooth surface that confines some tumors. I cut the specimen into two equal halves and realized that all of it, including the loose surface fragments, was tan-yellow tumor tissue. I submitted samples for microscopic study, including many designed to demonstrate the type of tissue on the surfaces. The tumor turned out to be a malignant tumor of fat tissue, called a liposarcoma. There is a spectrum of several types of this cancer, with a virtually benign variety at one end, and a highly malignant type at the other. This one was the worst kind. All of the microscopic sections demonstrated that the tissue on the surfaces, including both ends and around the middle of the mass, were pure liposarcoma with no hint of surrounding normal tissues. This meant that there was more malignant tumor tissue left behind in the surrounding tissues for unknown distances and with possible spread via the bloodstream to other organs such as the lungs and liver.

These findings made it necessary for the surgeon to operate again a few days later and cut out a generous portion of the chest wall, which he intended to be large enough to contain all of the remaining cancer. He excised an elliptical portion of the chest wall including the skin down to the rib cage measuring about 9 by 6 inches in greatest diameter. The size of the specimen, which also contained the sutured wound of the original operation along its center, gave reason to hope that the entire cancer was within it and that all of its surfaces were free of tumor. The microscopic sections taken of the sutured wound showed expected fields of residual cancer. To my horror, the section of the upper skin edge showed infiltrating liposarcoma, which extended right to the edge, indicating that residual tumor still remained in the patient. This finding also shook up the surgeon.

Dr. Harry M. Zimmerman, the head of the pathology department, contacted me after the surgeon sought his advice and asked to see the case prior to a meeting of the tumor board. It was customary for difficult cases to be referred to them for a consensus on further treatment. Dr. Zimmerman was a member of this board. I reviewed the case thoroughly with him, including the critical detail of the microscopic section showing the cancer right on the very edge of the specimen. One could see that the edges of the section corresponded exactly to the edges of the defect of the excised sample remaining in the specimen. This visualization of the tumor extending to the very edge left no doubt that residual cancer remained in the patient. The tumor board met and advised an even wider full thickness excision of the chest wall, including skin down to the rib cage, and using skin grafts from the thigh to cover the extensive defect. The recommended extent of the excision was from just below the armpit down to the lower rib margin.

This was done and the rectangular specimen measured about 12 by 8 inches with the sutured wound of the second operation in its center. I again studied samples of the center and all edges of the specimen and found no evidence of residual cancer. This did not mean that we were mistaken about the cancer extending to an edge of the previous specimen. Considering the fact that it would take about four thousand sections to see 1 cubic inch of tissue microscopically, the samples we studied represented a tiny microscopic view of the whole specimen. This specimen totaled more than 100 cubic inches, but it was still reassuring to find no tumor in our many samples.

I was saddened to learn that the tumor recurred in the right armpit three years later with spread to other organs. I brooded over this case during the three to four week hospital course and thereafter. I felt some guilt about being spared the pain of having to speak to the patient and his family. This was the difficult job of the surgeon, which I did not envy.

Guidelines to the management of soft tissue tumors were not well defined in those days because any one surgeon saw so few cases. Experiences with cases like this one led to a consensus about ideal management. Since all parts of the body are possible sites of these tumors, it became clear that the approach to radical surgery had to be planned in advance. The chance location of these tumors required a detailed study of the involved anatomy and the unique limitations to surgical excision a particular site might present. It became mandatory never to completely excise the tumor initially before carefully taking a biopsy through a small skin incision from the center of the tumor mass. The presence of the intact tumor was necessary at the time of radical surgery to enable the surgeon to plan an excision that would assure that all the surfaces of the specimen would consist of normal tissues with the cancer deep in its center. I always recall this case wondering how the patient would have fared if these guidelines had been followed.

6

How a Benign Tumor Can Kill

I was in the first year of my residency in pathology. This was one of my early autopsies and the first of endless surprises. The patient was a young woman in her late thirties who had a history of progressive heart failure[1], which began about a year before she was admitted. A diagnosis of stenosis of the mitral valve due to rheumatic heart disease had been established on physical examination, which revealed the typical heart murmur of this disease[2]. As sometimes happens, this patient did not have the usual history of acute rheumatic fever in childhood to account for having mitral stenosis as an adult. Some cases are apparently so mild in the early attacks as to escape notice even though each attack causes permanent injury to the heart and its valves. These silent cases surface when heart failure appears and causes symptoms like shortness of breath.

I began the postmortem study fully expecting to see an example of classical mitral stenosis. When I dissected the heart, I was startled to find that the mitral

---

1. See Appendix A.
2. The delicate mitral valve in the heart opens and closes with every heartbeat, an average of 72 beats per minute. When it opens, a batch of blood flows through it from the lungs into the left ventricle, which is the large left side of the heart. The heart then contracts for the next beat and the blood in the left ventricle is pumped out of the heart through another valve, called the aortic valve, to supply blood to all parts of the body. The open mitral valve is actually large enough for a ping-pong ball to pass through it.

    The valve is injured repeatedly in attacks of active rheumatic fever in childhood and adolescent years. The end result is a severely scarred and deformed valve with a rigid small slit-like opening no bigger than the buttonhole of a suit jacket. All of the blood circulating through the body has to trickle through this bottleneck. The blood dammed up behind the valve engorges the lungs first and then all the other organs causing difficulty in breathing, liver abnormalities, and difficulties in digestion. Death inevitably results when the obstruction causes insufficient blood flow to the brain. (See Appendix A).

valve was perfectly normal. The next shocker was the cause of the obstruction of the mitral valve. I found a tumor shaped like a ball as big as an average peach stuck to the inner surface of the chamber just above the valve. This chamber, called the left atrium[3], is where a batch of blood from the lungs accumulates before the valve opens and the blood pours through it into the left ventricle. I immediately realized that this was a classical example of how a benign tumor can kill by interfering with the mechanics of how organs work. Every medical student learns this principle with this example. The rare tumor is called a myxoma because of the sparse numbers of benign embryonic cells scattered in it and separated by a substance resembling Jell-O ®. This tumor literally acted as a ball-valve by obstructing blood flow during every heartbeat and by being pushed into the mitral valve opening by blood flowing into the left ventricle. The heart murmur of mitral stenosis, a typical sign of rheumatic heart disease, was exactly reproduced in this case by the partial obstruction of the valve by the overhanging tumor.

I experienced a delayed reaction of hopelessness when I realized our inadequacies of diagnosis and treatment at that time. These tumors were only visible on chest X-rays in exceptional cases, which showed areas of calcification outlining the tumor. Otherwise, they are lost in the shadows of the heart and its contents of blood. The other frustrating thing about it is that it would be so easy to cut it out, if there were a way to do it during life. It would be about ten years later when mechanical artificial hearts became practical to enable cutting the heart open during life and performing all sorts of cardiac surgery. Today, the imaging technology of ultrasound enables physicians to clearly view the inside of a beating heart and see its valves. This is a routine part of the examination of the heart and can easily reveal the tumor at an early stage when it can be excised surgically. In hindsight, I now realize that if I were immortal, there would be no end to the procession of such memorable cases.

---

3. See Appendix A.

7

How Fast Can a Cancer Grow?

One day in 1953, during my second year of training in pathology, a member of the tuberculosis service alerted me about a patient who was to have surgery the following day. The patient had tuberculosis and had been under treatment at our Bedford Sanatorium. The doctor showed me two chest X-rays. One was taken two days before admission to our hospital and the other a month before. These X-rays were the most recent of monthly X-rays taken routinely of all patients being treated at the sanatorium. Both X-rays showed the typical shadow of tuberculosis in a part of one lung. He pointed out that the only difference between the two was the presence of a small ovoid shadow the size of a small peanut in the more recent X-ray. It was in the center of the larger shadow of tuberculosis. This finding was very suspicious of a cancer developing within a site of tuberculosis, which does happen. One of the choices for the treatment of tuberculosis in those days was to simply cut out the diseased part of the lung. In this case, cutting out the whole lobe would treat both the infection and the tumor and provide a biopsy for microscopic study to determine whether or not it was malignant.

The surgery was performed by one of our excellent chest surgeons the next day. I quickly took the infectious specimen to the autopsy room and distended the lung with formaldehyde, which I injected into the cut end of its main bronchus. This sterilized the contagious lung and also prepared the tissues for microscopic study. I deliberately injected enough to distend the lung as it looks in inspiration. The following day, I carefully dissected open the main bronchus lengthwise and its smaller branches. I followed the small branch entering the diseased part and exposed an ovoid discrete white tumor growing in the bronchus and slightly distending it. The permanent microscopic slides were ready the next day, and it turned out to be the most malignant type of lung cancer called the small cell cancer, which refers to its microscopic appearance. I thought this was a therapeutic triumph because this tumor, which was diagnosed so early, had an optimal chance of cure. This type of cancer was well known as the most malignant and common type of lung cancer. I had admitted several men with it when I was an intern on the Neoplastic Service. These patients all seemed normal on admission, but they all had biopsy proven small cell cancers, which had already spread to other organs. They deteriorated rapidly with profound weight loss and died in less than three months.

Based on my past experience with this cancer, I was convinced that this patient might be the rare one that could be cured because it was discovered so early. Three months later, I was startled to learn that the patient died and was one of the cases being presented at our autopsy conference. The findings were typical of all patients with small cell cancer of the lung. The remaining lung showed a large recurrent growth of cancer, which spread to other organs including a liver weighing six pounds, or twice the normal weight, due to its additional load of cancer. I wondered how any case could be cured after seeing this one, and it eventually became common knowledge that a surgical cure was impossible.

My disenchantment with surgical treatment of this cancer was complete after I later autopsied a patient with widespread cancer in the brain and many other organs. The primary source of the cancer was unknown. Occasionally, the symptoms presented by patients with cancers are due to involvement of an organ to which the cancer spread, and the primary tumor may be silent. My main purpose in this case was to identify the source of the silent primary cancer. We discovered a tiny tumor in the lung having the typical microscopic features of a primary cancer arising in a very small bronchus, similar to the source in the case described above. This tiny cancer was less than ¼ inch in diameter and located just under the lung surface distant from the base of the lung. It was located at the end of a chain of four or five cancerous masses that got progressively larger up to the size of a walnut in the base of the lung. I never understood this growth pattern, but it was well known that tiny cancers could spread to other organs as huge tumors. The explanation is unknown.

Later studies by Dr. H. Coons at the M.D. Anderson Hospital in Houston, Texas, clarified my understanding of the behavior of this tumor. He devised a crude but informative way of understanding the growth of cancers. He took advantage of cancers whose diameters could be measured easily on X-rays at regular intervals. These included inoperable lung cancers or others that were never removed because the patients refused surgery. He determined the time it took for a cancer to double in size, or what became known as the doubling time. This was of no value in managing individual cases but was of value in understanding the behavior of different types of tumors. For example, X-ray studies of colon cancers revealed an average doubling time of six hundred days, in keeping with their relatively slow progression. The small cell lung cancer turned up with the fastest doubling time of two weeks. Consider what this means for the case I described. It was first seen as a tumor measuring about ½ inch in diameter. It would have measured 1 inch in two weeks, 2 inches in four weeks, 4 inches in six weeks, and 8 inches in eight weeks. Although the primary tumor was already removed, its spread had already occurred and grown at this rate. It was easy to understand why these unfortunate patients died in less than three months after the tumors were diagnosed.

This type of cancer was considered inoperable after many failures of surgical treatment throughout the country. However, the good news is that currently some of these cases are surviving for years. A combination of new chemical treatments for cancer and X-ray treatment of the brain and spinal cord is resulting in survivals for as many as ten years free of cancer.

8

Looks Aren't Everything

Physicians and patients are gratified by all the new discoveries in medical treatments that cure diseases and repair injuries. However, despite all these technological advances, Mother Nature is still indispensable because the work of restoring the normal structures of damaged organs is hers alone. This healing process is taken for granted, but successful treatments would be useless without it, and none can match the preeminence of Nature's role in healing. But while Nature is the unseen guardian angel in every patient-doctor encounter, She is also mischievous and enjoys fooling doctors by mimicry and by unexpected actions. Mimicry is well known in nature. Bitter-tasting butterflies discouraging predators are mimicked by look-alike tasty species. Harmless snakes mimic fearful poisonous ones with similar markings and behavior.

Nature also enjoys baffling us with completely unexpected signs and behaviors of diseases, which can lead us to a wrong diagnosis. I am reminded of lightning, which rarely occurs from a cloudless sky. The explanation is a horizontally propagated bolt from clouds beyond the horizon. The following case is an example of both mimicry and unexpected acts by a disease.

An internist friend visited me one day in 1957, my last year of training at Montefiore Hospital. He had a certain look in his eyes, a subtle smile that said "Gotcha," which alerted me to his presenting me with a tough problem. He first showed me a chest X-ray of his patient, a woman in her seventies. He obtained it one year before as part of an investigation of her vague complaints of not feeling well. The X-ray showed that both lungs contained about six to eight scattered tumors about the size of golf balls. He asked what I thought of it and I responded with an answer he expected, that it looked like a characteristic example of metastatic cancer to the lungs. In other words, these tumors had spread to the lungs from a primary cancerous source in some other organ. I also suggested that although any organ could be a possible source, the kidney was the most likely one because kidney cancers produce this X-ray picture of lungs more consistently than cancers from other organs.

He agreed with my statement, and showed me a subsequent X-ray study of the kidneys, which did not reveal the expected kidney cancer. Only a microscopic study of a biopsy of the tumors in the lung would suggest its actual source. Sure enough, the internist then produced the microscopic slide of the biopsy taken the year before of one of the tumors in the lung. I eagerly examined the slide expecting a surprise of some sort. Although the X-rays of the kidneys failed to reveal any cancer, the tumors in the lungs turned out to be a typical example of a common cancer of the kidney called a "clear cell carcinoma."

Lack of any evidence of a primary tumor of the kidney then prompted the physicians to examine other organs, which could all produce tumors infrequently having the identical microscopic appearance of a "clear cell carcinoma." The other suspect organs included the adrenal glands, ovaries and salivary glands, which were investigated.

X-ray studies showed no evidence of tumors in either adrenal gland, which are located immediately above the kidneys. An examination of the pelvic organs by palpation revealed two ovaries of normal size with no evidence of a tumor. A tumor of salivary gland origin was ruled out by simple physical examination, which revealed no evidence of swelling of the face in front of the ears or under the jaws, where two large salivary glands are located. Nothing more could be done and the patient was then followed for further developments.

All of the concerned physicians expected progression of cancerous spread in the lungs and to other organs. There was a possibility that the primary source would eventually reveal itself by new symptoms and signs, although occasionally patients die with disseminated spread of cancers without an obvious primary source. Autopsies will usually reveal the site of origin, but there are rare cases where the source is not found.

I listened expectantly to my friend's continuing story because there were clearly more surprises to come since everything he related happened the year before. Like a magician pulling a rabbit out of a hat, he produced a second more astounding surprise, a current chest X-ray, which looked completely normal. All the tumors, which were seen and biopsied the year before, had disappeared! It was unbelievable. All of us, including the head of pathology, Dr. H.M. Zimmerman, were now baffled. Dr. Zimmerman asked me to send the biopsy slides to Dr. Arthur Purdy Stout[1], who suggested that this might not be a cancer at all but rather a benign fat storage disease[2]. A colleague of Dr. Stout, Dr. Oscar Auerbach[3], who was an authority on lung diseases, also saw the case and offered the same opinion. We had no other way of explaining this mystery and accepted the opinions of the two experts, because the appearance of immune cells containing fat and looking exactly like clear cell cancer of the kidney was well known.

Later that year, I joined the staff of the Jewish Hospital of St. Louis, an affiliate of Washington University, as the Director of Pathology and Laboratories. I visited Montefiore Hospital in New York one year later and met my internist friend in the corridors. After exchanging greetings, he immediately refreshed my memory about this case and hit me with the third surprise when he related that the patient developed painless bleeding into the urine a few months earlier. This is a characteristic symptom of many things, including a cancer of the kidney. This time, routine X-ray studies of the kidneys did reveal an obvious tumor on one side. It was removed and was a typical clear cell carcinoma. The chest X-ray was still free of spread of the cancer. We discussed the case and agreed that it was likely that the tumor was too small to be seen on the initial kidney X-rays two years before. But we were both puzzled by the appearance of the tumors in the lungs, and their magical disappearance without any treatment. The primary cancer in the kidney continued to grow for at least two years, during the same time that its earlier cancerous spread to the lungs simply disappeared.

The spontaneous regression of cancers is a rare phenomenon that has since been seen with other cancers but more often with kidney cancer. This case was my only personal experience with this behavior. A possible cause for this was unknown then and now. Today, a reasonable explanation may be the role of our immune system in combating cancer, which remains to be seen. It is interesting that experimental methods of treating cancer today include stimulating the immune system by deliberately injecting a foreign protein into the patient. The

---

1. Dr. Arthur Purdy Stout was the most renowned surgical pathologist of his time because of his many contributions. He was chief of surgical pathology at the Presbyterian Hospital in New York, the University Hospital of Columbia's College of Physicians and Surgeons.
2. There are many different kinds of fat that are components of different organs. For example, the fats that are unique for the brain are different from the familiar fat of obesity. A specific type of fat accumulates in cells of the immune system in each of the rare storage diseases sufficient to form discreet tumors made up of immune cells loaded with fat. The problem is that these benign fat-laden immune cells can sometimes look like a clear cell carcinoma under the microscope (See Appendix B).
3. Dr. Oscar Auerbach was the renowned leading investigator of the group that included Dr. Stout and that presented the first hard evidence that smoking caused lung cancer in 1957.

theory is that a stimulated immune system would be more effective in attacking a cancer. This was a humbling experience for every involved doctor.

Technological progress would have made the diagnostic management of this case less perplexing if it happened today. The CAT scan and MRI might very well identify early cancers that might be missed on routine X-rays. There is also now a microscopic chemical test that easily distinguishes this type of kidney cancer from a look-alike fat storage disease.

I do not know the final outcome of this patient's story. One possibility is that she remained free of cancer and died of some other disease. The more likely possibility is that she died of eventual spread to other organs. This could occur many years after surgery. I once autopsied an elderly man in his late 80s who died of a recurrence of a kidney cancer in the bed of the removed kidney thirty-seven years after the operation. Here again, the immune system may have had a role in suppressing the growth of viable remaining nests of cancer.

1957–66, The Jewish Hospital of St. Louis, Missouri, Director of Laboratories

9

Managing an Insoluble Problem

Practicing doctors often regard pathologists as sages who have privileged access to knowledge unknown to others. They expect answers to questions that no one can answer because of vast voids in our knowledge. A popular quip, "Surgeons know nothing and do everything, and pathologists know everything and do nothing," reflects their image of pathologists. They have utmost confidence in our ability to make correct diagnoses on all biopsies of diseased tissues. This confidence is usually justified because we are very good at this. But we also have to cope with uncertainty, which they usually find very distressing because we then fail to help them. Just as Mother Nature makes atypical varieties of diseases, which are sometimes misdiagnosed, atypical varieties of disease manifestations occur in tissues, which we either cannot diagnose on microscopic study or which can even mislead us to a wrong diagnosis.

A revealing early example of our limitations occurred to me in 1958. A man in his mid-thirties had developed a recurrent tumor in his femur, the long bone in the thigh between the hip and knee joints. His medical history indicated that, about two years ago, a continuous pain in his thigh prompted him to see a doctor. An X-ray revealed a tumor about the size of a peach pit in the lower end of the femur, approximately 6 inches above the knee joint. The tumor occupied the soft central marrow cavity and was sharply outlined. An orthopedic surgeon operated and scooped out as much of the tumor as possible using a curette, which is a rigid steel instrument with a handle connected to a small spoon, less than ½ inch in diameter. All of the tumor fragments were sent to the pathologist for microscopic study. The tumor was made up of normal looking cartilaginous tissue suggesting one of two possibilities. The most likely diagnosis was a benign cartilaginous tumor, which was the diagnosis reported. The other remote possibility was a malignant cartilaginous tumor, which would require an amputation to prevent the spread of the cancer to the rest of the body.

How can a benign looking tumor turn out to be malignant? The answer is that malignancy is also determined by the subsequent behavior of some tumors. For example, there are tumors that look malignant under microscopic study and are easily cured by simply cutting them out without any further worry about the tumor spreading to other organs. There are also tumors that look benign and have a nasty habit of spreading like cancers anyhow. Fortunately, such tumors are well known and anticipated by pathologists. A benign looking cartilaginous tumor in this location occasionally does behave as a malignant tumor. The pathologist, who diagnosed this case as benign, made a diligent microscopic study of it looking for evidence of early malignancy, yet found none and decided on a benign diagnosis.

Pain in the thigh recurred two years later. An X-ray revealed several pea-sized foci of tumor around the peripheral margins of the original tumor. This was a recurrence of the tumor arising from microscopic islands left behind during the original excision. This actually can happen and is not entirely preventable no matter how vigorously the surgeon scraped out the original tumor because microscopic islands can get into the spongy surrounding bone beyond the reach of the curette.

Now the chips were down and the question was to assume it was still benign and curette out more tissue for study or to do an amputation. The orthopedist was in a bind because it was impossible to get out the entire recurrent tumor with a curette. If a few biopsies were taken and all appeared benign, this would still not guarantee benign behavior. A review of the original biopsies was in order, which I did painstakingly and searched for any evidence of malignancy that would justify an amputation. Like the previous pathologist, I could not find a hint of malignant changes.

The orthopedist had received his specialty training at the Hospital for Joint Diseases in New York City and studied bone diseases under Dr. Henry Jaffee[1]. He suggested that I send the slides to his esteemed professor for a consultation. The questions put to Dr. Jaffee were whether or not the tumor was malignant and if uncertain, whether to proceed with an amputation. Dr. Jaffe's response made me realize how dark a shadow uncertainty can cast on pathology. He indicated that it could be malignant even though it looked benign and that its future

---

1. Dr. Henry Jaffee was the chief pathologist at the Hospital for Joint Diseases in New York City. He was then the leading authority on bone tumors in the United States, pioneering the original descriptions of several varieties of bone tumors and writing the major reference book on the subject.

behavior was unpredictable. He could not recommend or criticize amputation and left the decision up to the orthopedist.

The orthopedist ultimately decided on an alternative action, which I had not realized was possible. He decided to cut out the portion of the femur containing the recurrent tumors, and fuse the remaining two cut ends of the femur to one another, resulting in a shortened bone. This action resulted in a shortened leg, which was preferable to amputation. The specimen was a 3- to 4-inch segment of femur with the lesions in its center and both cut margins made up of normal bone and marrow. I was able to examine the several recurrent tumors and they all looked as benign as the original ones.

As a young pathologist, I always sensed the need to be as positive as possible about my diagnoses, in order to earn the confidence of doctors referring cases to me. I dreaded the cases with uncertain diagnoses, which opened my credibility to question. My experience with Dr. Jaffee taught me a frustrating reality. The admission of uncertainty by an average pathologist immediately cast doubt on his credibility, which could only be restored by an authority having the same uncertainty. Other authoritative pathologists, like Drs. Arthur Purdy Stout and Lauren V. Ackerman, were indispensable for the solution of diagnostic problems of rare or first-of-kind cases, which appear sporadically with little or no information in the books about them. Their consultations provided the best judgments possible to intelligent decisions on treatments. The ultimate resource for such service in the United States was and still is the Armed Forces Institute of Pathology (AFIP) in Washington, DC. They serve all the U.S. army and naval hospitals in the world and see an enormous number of cases. The members of their staff are experts in various types of tumors and infectious diseases. Their strength is further enhanced by the fact that authorities throughout the country in medical centers are often consultants to the AFIP.

In this case, Dr. Henry Jaffee's response was, "I don't know." He also declined a recommendation for or against amputation. I never again received an identical response from any other consultant in more than forty years. There have been rare instances of the behavior of a tumor proving a consultant's diagnosis wrong. The fact is that nature does not spare consultants of limitations anymore than the rest of us. They do the best they can in problem cases by taking into account the possible diagnoses and the quality of life concerns of minor versus radical surgery. There are inevitable insoluble cases and perhaps the best approach to deciding management is to present the facts to patients and learn their wishes.

10

A Humiliating Mistake

This incident occurred in the early months after I joined the Jewish Hospital of St. Louis. My reputation preceded me in autopsy pathology and I sensed the confidence that internists had in my diagnoses from the start. My consultations with surgeons in the operating room and the numerous reports I issued on biopsies enhanced my credibility as a surgical pathologist. I introduced a weekly surgical pathology conference featuring biopsies and frozen sections with diagnostic problems in order to firmly establish my credibility. I called this conference a "goof conference" because it included all cases with any differences between diagnoses I made in the operating room and in final reports.

The pathology department at Montefiore Hospital did not have this type of conference. I learned about it from one of my classmates, Dr. Howard Dorfman, who trained under Dr. Arthur Purdy Stout, the head of surgical pathology at the Presbyterian Hospital in New York. Dr. Stout was then considered the top American surgical pathologist and ran a weekly popular "goof conference."

This conference served several purposes. It put to rest all rumors about any possible errors that may have been committed. It reviewed all frozen sections with diagnoses that I postponed until I could see better permanent slides. Most importantly, this conference educated the surgeons about the limitations of frozen sections. For example, there is a sampling limitation of frozen sections, which reduces diagnostic accuracy. Consider a frozen section of a lymph node, in search of any evidence of spread of a cancer. A negative result is good news, justifying surgery in an attempt to cure. An inevitable problem, however, is that the permanent sections may reveal a microscopic island of cancerous spread, which was not seen in the frozen section. Invariably, a comparison of the frozen and permanent sections projected on a screen for all to see clearly proved that the frozen section simply showed no evidence of cancerous spread. The sampling limitation is that the frozen section is one tiny slice out of a possible five hundred thin slices that can be prepared from one biopsy specimen. This introduces the inherent inaccuracy of the frozen section, due to the fact that there is no guarantee that the slices from rest of the block of specimen, remaining for permanent sections, will be free of cancer. The conference was also valuable because of the exposure of medical students and trainees to pathology in action.

The obvious downside of this conference was the exposure of my limitations, which were as inevitable for me as any physician. Diagnostic mistakes happen and command more attention in such a conference than any other subject. The fact is that the educational value of these misdiagnosed cases was incalculable and actually contributed to my credibility. The following incident is a tale of one of my "goofs," which did not involve a frozen section.

One of the diagnostic problems pathologists had in the early days was distinguishing between benign and malignant polyps of the large intestine. Benign polyps are common and occasionally can develop into cancers. The appearance of stools stained with blood is a common symptom of a bleeding benign polyp, but may also be due to hemorrhoids, a malignant polyp or a frank cancer. Today, a bleeding source can be found with a colonoscope, which is equipped to excise polyps. It is a tubular flexible instrument, which is inserted into the rectum under light anesthesia and fed through the entire large intestine (colon) in order to visualize its inner surface.

Prior to the invention of the colonoscope about thirty years ago, only polyps in the lower colon and rectum could be visualized and excised with a sigmoidoscope, a rigid tubular instrument inserted into the rectum. X-ray studies utilizing a barium enema facilitated the location of polyps higher in the colon, which were easily seen because the barium solution coated the polyps making them visible on X-rays.

The patient was a young woman in her forties with blood-stained stools. Examination of the lower colon and rectum with a sigmoidoscope was negative. A barium enema revealed a polyp higher in the colon about the size of a seeded grape. An operation was performed and the polyp was easily snipped off from the inner wall of the colon. The polyp looked benign to the naked eye and, as usual, had a short stalk like a mushroom. The microscopic appearance of the polyp revealed an early cancer on its surface. This immediately posed a problem, which was unresolved at that time. The problem was whether to proceed with a radical removal of more of the colon, including regional lymph nodes that might contain islands of cancer, or to do nothing.

There were two schools of thought at the time. The more popular one was the result of the individual experiences of many surgeons, who realized that the patients did fine with no further treatment when an early cancer was confined to the surface of a polyp. The other viewpoint was driven by the conviction that early cancers can spread early and required the same radical surgery as any other cancer.

The choice of treatment was up to the surgeon and the patient, and the decision was to proceed with a radical removal of more colon with regional lymph nodes. My examination of the colon was completely negative. The critical part of the examination was to determine whether the cancerous focus in the polyp had spread to the lymph nodes. This was important because the outlook for a cure was almost 100% if the lymph nodes were spared. I carefully dissected more than a dozen lymph nodes from the specimen and studied them all microscopically. I was surprised to find microscopic glands in one lymph node that looked like abnormal colon glands. I had to conclude that this was an early case of focal cancer in an otherwise benign polyp that actually did spread to the lymph nodes.

The roof fell in. My finding spread throughout the surgical department because this was big news, a case with proven spread of a focal cancer in a polyp to lymph nodes. Eventually, the word spread to the university hospital and their pathology department, and I was asked to show the case to them. I did so and experienced the first of a few humiliating and regretful experiences of my career as a pathologist. A sympathetic gynecologist who specialized in gynecological pathology reviewed the slide with me and pointed out that the glands in the lymph node did not come from the polyp or any part of the colon. The glands were benign glands that came from the inner lining of the uterus called the endometrium. This is the tissue that is normally passed out with every menstrual period in the absence of an early pregnancy. I looked at it with him under the high power of the microscope and was embarrassed to see the numerous little hairs on the surfaces of these cells, which clearly identified them as benign endometrial cells. This patient had an obscure disease called endometriosis, which is not rare. It is characterized by islands of benign endometrial tissues in pelvic organs entirely separate from the uterus. The islands can be found in the ovaries, fallopian tubes, wall of the colon or in lymph nodes. It is still a mystery as to how they get to these sites, but they are not cancerous. They even degenerate and bleed with every menstrual cycle. This causes complications due to the effects of these repeated hemorrhages in odd places. An important complication is sterility due to blocked involved fallopian tubes as a result of scarring following repeated small hemorrhages. Dr. Lauren V. Ackerman was then the director of Surgical Pathology at Barnes Hospital and an internationally recognized leader in his field after publishing his famous textbook, which is still a major reference. He presented this case at the university hospital because of its teaching value to an audience of medical students, surgeons and pathologists. This case was of great interest, due to the fact that no one up to that time had been able to demonstrate that surface cancers in otherwise benign colonic polyps could spread to lymph nodes. Furthermore, the case illustrated another pitfall in diagnostic pathology, mistaking a benign process as a cancer. One young surgeon criticized my error as inexcusable and asked where the case originated. To my relief, Dr. Ackerman declined to reveal the source. But I agreed with that young surgeon, because I could not tolerate any error as a young pathologist because of my conviction that all errors were avoidable. I eventually realized thirty years later that unavoidable errors do indeed occur in medical practice.

11

A Pathologist's Nightmare

This story requires basic knowledge of the anatomy and purpose of the pancreas in order to understand the Whipple operation. This is a challenging surgical technique named after its originator and is a radical operation to remove a cancer of the pancreas.

The pancreas is situated in the center of the abdomen behind the stomach and below the liver. See Figure 1.

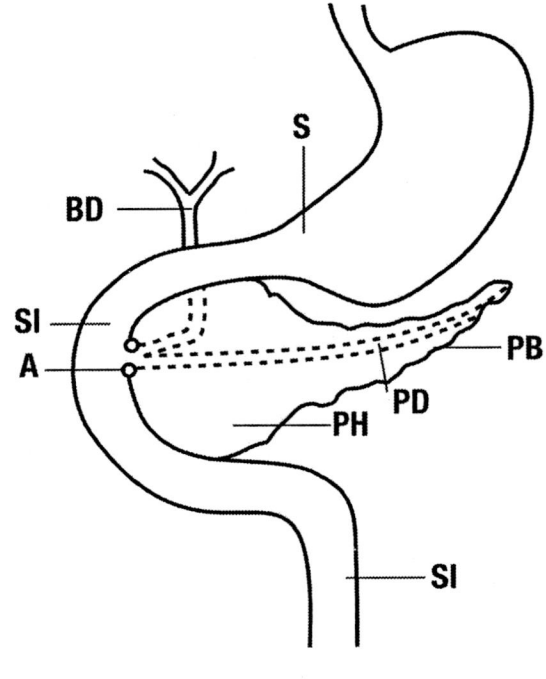

Figure 1

It is shaped like a tadpole with a head (Fig. 1 PH) on the right side and a body and tail, which extend to the left (Fig. 1 PB). It is a major source of digestive juices, which flow from the pancreatic duct (Fig. 1 PD) into the upper end of the small intestines (Fig. 1 SI) below its junction with the lower end of the stomach (Fig. 1 S) through a small nipple-like opening in its wall called the ampulla (Fig. 1 A). The pancreas also contains thousands of microscopic glands, which produce insulin, a hormone that maintains a normal sugar concentration in the blood and is used to treat diabetes. The head is about the size of a hamburger, which is attached along its right margin to the small intestine at the ampulla and rests on a large artery and vein behind, which is the main blood supply to the intestines. The liver produces bile, which is also necessary for digestion. The bile duct (Fig. 1 BD) brings bile to the small intestine through the ampulla where it joins the pancreatic duct. The lower end of the small intestine (Fig. 1 SI) continues for twenty-five feet to its junction with the large intestine.

The Whipple operation is used to remove the head of the pancreas containing a cancer, which may arise in the pancreas itself or in the ampulla. The difference between the two possible sites of origin is important because the Whipple operation cures most cancers of the ampulla and only a small percentage of cancers within the head of the pancreas. Cancers of the pancreas arising in the body or tail are rarely treated surgically because the first symptom of this silent cancer is usually caused by spread to other organs. The operation requires that the surgeon must do four transections of major organs in order to remove the head of the pancreas and the loop of small intestine adherent to the right margin of the head where the ampulla enters it. See Figure 2.

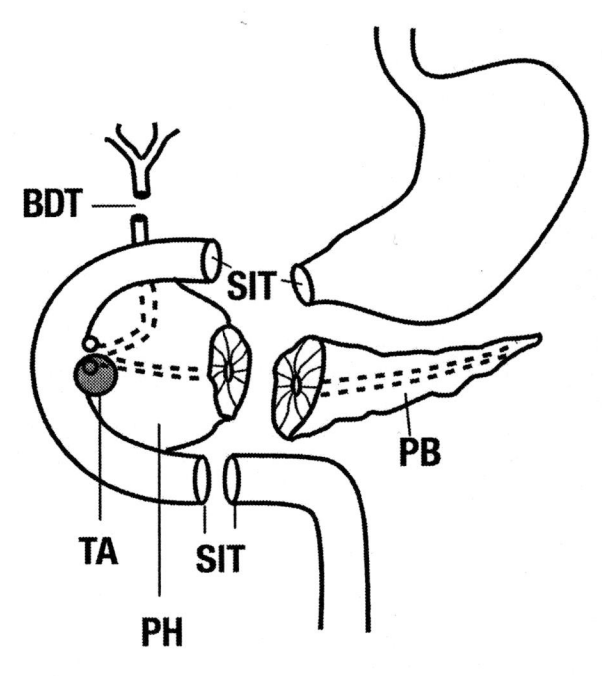

Figure 2

Two transections are made across the small intestine, one above the head (Fig. 2 SIT) where the stomach joins the beginning of the small intestine and one below the head (Fig. 2 SIT) where the remainder of some twenty-five feet of small intestine begins. The bile duct is transected just above the head (Fig. 2 BDT) and a final transection is made across the junction of the head and body of the pancreas (Fig. 2 PB). The head of the pancreas (Fig. 2 PH) is then removed with the tumor of the ampulla (Fig. 2 TA).

The surgeon achieves reconstruction by mobilizing the upper end of the small intestine and manipulating a loop to set up the following restorations. See Figure 3.

A Pathologist's Nightmare 53

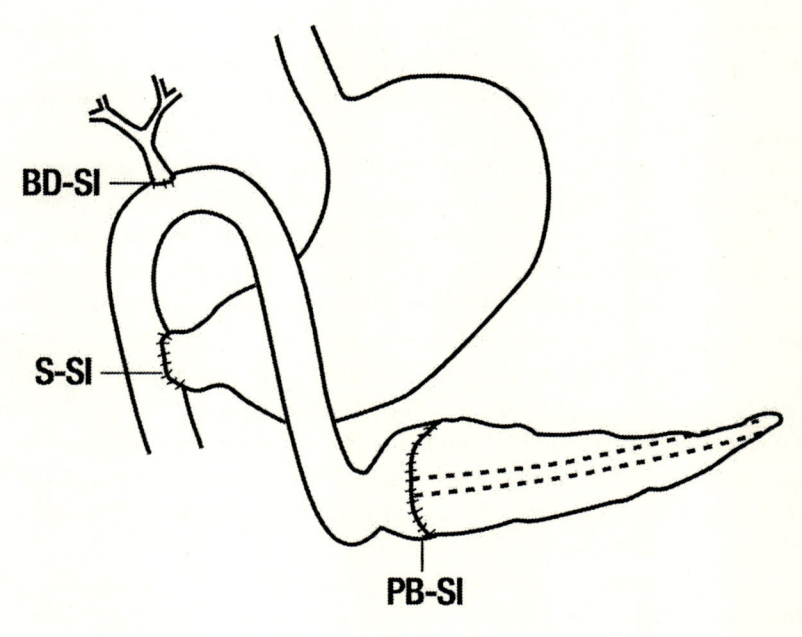

Figure 3

He joins the cut open end of the small intestine to the raw cut surface of the pancreatic body (Fig. 3 PB-SI) thus restoring the entry of pancreatic digestive juices. He joins the open end of the stomach to the side of the loop of small intestine thus restoring flow of stomach contents into it (Fig. 3 S-SI). The cut end of the bile duct is similarly joined to the side of the small intestinal loop (Fig. 3 BD-SI) and the procedure is completed.

In 1957 I had been at the Jewish Hospital of Saint Louis for a few months and had become friendly with the surgical residents, who were a little younger than me. They were all very bright and were carefully selected from the best candidates by our chief of surgery. I was called to the operating room one day by one of the assistant residents who I liked very much. He was very friendly and bashful, acting more like a medical student than a surgical resident. He was raised on a farm in Hannibal, Missouri—Mark Twain country—and he behaved like a typical "country boy." Another resident assisted him and a member of the attending staff stood by as a supervisor. He presented me with a biopsy of a tumor of the ampulla of the pancreas and asked if I would do a frozen section.[1] I took a portion of the biopsy for frozen section. The entire specimen was pure tumor tissue without any adherent normal tissue. The cells appeared suspicious of a cancer but could also still be a benign tumor. I had to see the border between the tumor and surrounding tissues to see whether the tumor cells invaded normal tissues, which was proof of malignancy. I told the surgeon what I thought, which included the comment that it was probably malignant, expecting him to end the procedure and wait until the next day for a final answer before any definitive surgery.

He called me back to the operating room four hours later and a nurse handed me a Whipple specimen (Fig. 2) on a tray. I was shocked out of my wits. The resident looked up and quietly said, "Well, there it is. I thought you might want to start working on it now because I know it will take some time." I was speechless and left the operating room absolutely stunned. My only exposure to the Whipple operation was to hear it discussed at conferences concerning surgical treatment for cancer of the pancreas at Montefiore Hospital. Although frequently mentioned, I never knew of any case being done there during my training. This was not surprising because the mortality rate of the operation was 25% and only 2% of the patients with cancer benefited from the operation. The others died from the spread of the cancer to other organs.

I brought the specimen to my laboratory and gazed at it in disbelief. There was the round head of the pancreas and the raw surface on its left side where it was cut from the body. A segment of small bowel, about 4 inches long, was attached to its right margin. I cut open this segment lengthwise to expose its inner lining and saw the tumor forming a grape-sized mass in the ampulla. The cut end of the obstructed and distended bile duct was easily seen just above the upper margin of the head. I dissected further and could see that the tumor involved obstructed both the bile and the pancreatic ducts at the ampulla. I prepared several microscopic sections to study the junction of the tumor and surrounding normal looking tissues for evidence of invasion. I had to wait to see these slides until the next day because the samples required automatic processing overnight.

I was tortured that night by a recurring nightmare. I found myself hoping that the sections would show invasion to justify such a radical operation, and was then overwhelmed by guilt for having such a wish. By morning, I made myself a sol-

---

1. A frozen section is a very thin slice of a frozen biopsy specimen, which is stained and studied microscopically by a pathologist during surgery. The purpose is to give the surgeon a rapid diagnosis, which enables an appropriate operation. A thin slice of frozen specimen is cut in a deep freezer with a slicer called a microtome, which is similar to a meat slicer in a delicatessen. The big difference is that frozen sections are extremely thin. One can prepare one-hundred frozen sections from a specimen, which measures 1/20th of an inch in thickness.

emn vow never again in my life to diagnose a frozen section as a cancer, without seeing decisive proof, or if there was a chance of any doubt or second thoughts. My criterion for the diagnosis of a cancer from a frozen section from that day forward was crystal clear. I must have absolute confidence in the diagnosis to the extent that my seeing the slides the next day would not be the cause for anxiety, but a necessary chore for a complete report. This case reminded me of an old saying in surgical pathology that was taught by my teacher, Dr. H.M. Zimmerman, "If there is any doubt, the answer is no."

The following morning, microscopic sections did show evidence of invasion. I was, of course, relieved. I recently contacted my friend, the surgeon who performed the operation, to learn what happened thereafter. I was very pleased and not surprised that the patient did well postoperatively and left the hospital without any further problems. I was not surprised because I eventually realized that the quality of surgery in Saint Louis was the best I had ever seen.

But there is more to this tale. I visited the Mayo Clinic in Rochester, Minnesota, about one year later in order to observe and learn their frozen section technique. I was curious and excited, because more than one surgeon at our hospital told me that frozen sections were done on all tissues at the Mayo Clinic. I had to see this for myself because I was sure they were exaggerating. Frozen sections were usually scheduled in advance, especially in small community hospitals that were served by iterant pathologists who served a network of hospitals on a part-time basis. The surgeons claimed that frozen sections were routine at the Mayo Clinic on specimens that I considered too difficult to prepare, such as polyps of the large intestine and the thyroid gland.

I wrote to the head of surgical pathology at the Mayo Clinic, Dr. Malcolm Dockerty, and asked if I could observe their technique. His response was the first of many pleasant surprises because he not only agreed but also expressed pleasure, as if I were the one granting a favor by visiting his facility. The visit to the Mayo Clinic turned out to be one of my most eye-opening experiences.

The Mayo Clinic is a modest title for a huge institution, because I had always thought of a clinic as a department in a hospital. The institution included two hospitals; the 900-plus bed Saint Mary's Hospital, the 300-plus bed Methodist Hospital and numerous motels in town, which also served as convalescent homes. The average length of stay in the hospitals was three days, compared to ten days at the Jewish Hospital of Saint Louis, which was about the national average at that time. They managed to limit the stay of postoperative cases by moving uncomplicated cases into the motels, where they continued to be seen regularly by visiting nurses and physicians. They were treated as in a hospital setting, including intravenous fluids. I was very impressed by this system, which made their productivity and income three times higher than the national average.

Dr. Dockerty kept me by his side all day as he performed his duties. We spent the morning at the Methodist Hospital, which contained an elaborate surgical pathology laboratory in the operating room complex. They had six individually manned frozen section benches compared to the one bench at the Jewish Hospital of Saint Louis where I made my own sections. Six technicians worked at each bench sectioning all the specimens. These included the urgent cases for deciding surgical procedures, and all others for routine studies and reports. Dr. Dockerty personally diagnosed every urgent frozen section, and I reveled in the excitement by looking at everything he did. At first, as I watched the technicians do their sections, I couldn't believe what they did. They instantly shaved a thin section from a frozen piece of tissue with a special knife and got it neatly on a slide with no wrinkles. It was a very rapid motion unlike my own, which was slow and always ending with annoying wrinkles. By the end of the day, I was doing sections like one of their technicians by benefiting from two requirements. One was a perfectly sharpened knife, provided by a department that made and maintained surgical instruments every day. The other was a maneuver they used to cut a section, which I would never have tried without seeing it work.

He drove me over to the Saint Mary's Hospital after a quick lunch, where I beheld a much bigger pathology laboratory in the operating room complex. They had twelve busy frozen section benches, and the afternoon passed quickly with intriguing cases and the continuous educational commentary of Dr. Dockerty, who I came to admire as a great teacher. I saw the progress of one case that was very revealing of their capabilities. It was a woman in her forties who had a prior biopsy of the uterine cervix, which showed a possibly invasive cancerous change. The choice was whether to just do a local excision of the cervix if there was no evidence of invasive cancer, or to then perform a radical removal of the uterus, fallopian tubes, ovaries and local glands if there was.

Such a study of the entire cervix was time consuming and usually required a thorough study of good permanent sections, which needed to wait till the following day. Dr. Dockerty reviewed all the frozen sections of the excised cervix within minutes and did find an invasive cancer, which justified a radical operation. Later, the specimen was thoroughly examined by other pathologists, who took the usual samples for microscopic study totaling some twenty frozen sections. They issued a completed report, which was in the patient's hospital chart before she left the operating room. It would have taken me two to three days to issue a similar report at my hospital.

Another feature of the streamlined medical care at the Mayo Clinic was specialization. I got the impression that just about any kind of surgery was done by near perfectionists in their field. I was reminded of their expertise a few years later when President Lyndon Johnson needed his gall bladder removed, which is a routine simple operation. Although there was a competent staff at the Walter Reed Army Hospital, he elected to fly in the whole team from the Mayo Clinic for the operation. After being overwhelmed by Dr. Dockerty and the incredible facilities, I developed a lasting impression that the Mayo Clinic was a medical paradise, where medicine was practiced the way one wished it were practiced everywhere.

When activities quieted down towards the end of that memorable day, and I looked up to Dr. Dockerty as a leader in his field, I was curious to learn how he managed to tell the difference between cancers and benign tumors of the ampulla of the pancreas in frozen sections. His answer was an example of one way we deal with uncertainty. He declared that you couldn't tell the difference on frozen section because the answer in many cases was dependent on the presence or absence of invasion of the surrounding normal tissues. As a practical matter, this means you have to examine the head of the pancreas around the ampulla and there is only one way to get enough of the head to study—the Whipple operation. He said all of these cases were diagnosed as malignant for this reason and that this is also justified by the extreme rarity of the benign cases. I heaved an inner sigh of relief when I realized that my blunder in suggesting that the frozen section of a tumor was malignant without proof turned out to be the right way to manage this tumor. The valuable lesson of this case was still intact, namely, to be sure that a tumor is a cancer before reporting it. Today, the mortality of the Whipple operation is extremely low and benefits about 25% of cases with cancers of the pancreas and 98% of those with tumors of the ampulla.

The frozen section has enriched the status of the operating room as a classroom, especially in a teaching hospital. The popularity of frozen sections increased to the point of surgeons expecting them for all types of specimens. It gives them instant answers, which makes them more comfortable in a stressful situation, and it is also a wonderful educational experience for attentive assistants and students.

12

Wow! A New Disease!

Introduction—What is an infarct?

This story requires an understanding of one way that organs suffering injury need medical attention. An occlusion of an artery supplying a portion of an organ results in death of the deprived tissues. The dead portion is called an infarct. The most common cause of death in our society is a loss of blood supply to the heart muscle, or the brain. The loss of blood supply is due to the disease called arteriosclerosis. This disease leads to the accumulation of fats and scar tissue in the walls of arteries, which gradually constricts blood flow to the point of complete obstruction. Infarcts of the heart wall, which range in size from microscopic proportions to those large enough to see with the naked eye at autopsy, are the basis for the common "heart attack."

A similar variation in severity occurs in the brain. An infarct can involve one whole side of the brain due to the occlusion of a major artery and be fatal. Smaller infarcts result in the common "stroke" from which patients often recover completely. Some patients are left with permanent paralysis and problems with speech. Infarcts of the intestine may occur, as well as infarcts of the legs, which usually require amputation due to gangrene.

The Patient's Story

One day in 1958, I performed an autopsy on an 87-year-old man, who was a resident in a nursing home. He was admitted because of severe abdominal pain and shock of several hours duration. Urgent studies were done to find the cause. An X-ray of the abdomen was taken immediately to see if there was free air in the abdominal cavity caused by a hole in the wall of the intestine, allowing intestinal contents and air to escape into the free abdominal cavity. This is a surgical emergency because repairing the hole is lifesaving. The results of X-rays ruled out the presence of free air, as well as of gallstones, another possible cause of severe abdominal pain. Acute inflammation of the pancreas called pancreatitis was another potentially deadly cause. Acute pancreatitis causes the concentration in the blood of a protein that it normally produces to sharply rise tenfold. This patient's blood test was normal, which eliminated pancreatitis as a possible diagnosis.

An infarct of the intestines was the remaining possibility. Normally, after partial digestion in the stomach, the intestinal contents pass into about 25 feet of small intestine for completion of digestion and absorption of nutrients, and then pass into about 5 feet of large intestine, where water is absorbed from the contents, forming solid feces. Intestinal infarcts are usually fatal because the occlusion is usually in a main artery that supplies blood to the entire small intestine and half of the large intestine. Surgical removal of the dead bowel would be easy, but this operation is useless since it is impossible to replace small intestinal function, which is essential for life. Occasional cases are more fortunate when the extent of the dead intestine is limited and easily removed surgically with survival because sufficient intact bowel remains for normal function.

With this possibility in mind, physicians relieved the patient's pain and applied remedies to treat shock in preparation for an emergency surgical exploration of the intestines to determine the exact extent of the infarct. The patient went deeper into shock despite all measures and went into a coma, which indicated that he probably had the usual deadly type of infarct. He died the day after admission and a consent for autopsy was obtained from the nearest of kin.

The autopsy presented me with a series of unexpected surprises. There were infarcts of the intestine but this was no ordinary extent of dead bowel, with live bowel above and below the infracted segment. There wasn't one infarct but many scattered throughout the small and large intestines, involving most of the bowel with random segments of living bowel between the infracted ones. The crazy distribution was unrelated to the distribution of any one occluded artery. I was then startled to find that half of the stomach was infracted. This was incredible because infarcts of the stomach are not supposed to happen because of its unusually rich blood supply from several arteries. The next surprise was the first infarct of the liver that I had ever seen. This is known to occur rarely and is usually due to a rare disease of the arteries called polyarteritis nodosa[1], unrelated to arteriosclerosis.

My dissection of the blood supply to all of the abdominal organs revealed only a mild degree of arteriosclerosis but no occlusions. I then began to suspect polyarteritis nodosa because of the random distribution of multiple infarcts in abdominal organs. The diagnostic features of this disease can only be found microscopically and I pursued this possibility. My exhaustive study of numerous samples of tissues was completely negative and I was baffled. Then it occurred to me that arsenic and mercury poisoning could result in death of tissues indistinguishable from infarcts. Chemical analyses of blood and tissue samples were negative for these poisons.

I was mystified at this point, which goes with the territory of all medical practice including pathology. These occasions remind us that there are vast voids in our knowledge and that Nature delights in confounding us by not reading our books on the way diseases are supposed to behave. Nature is very creative and her choices are endless.

I soon realized that others were as baffled as I was, when similar cases began to be reported in our medical journals. Physicians are often skeptical of the findings of a pathologist when an unfavorable result clashes with their mistaken diagnosis. The usual criticism, which is justified sometimes, is that the pathologist failed to find something that was surely there. It was this criticism that led to a series of events that initiated the ultimate solution to the cause of this disease. A bright resident in pathology at the Massachusetts General Hospital had autopsied a similar case and found no arterial occlusions. The chief of surgery flatly told the resident that he must have missed it. The resident was affronted and seized his opportunity for satisfaction when another subsequent autopsy showed a similar unusual distribution of intestinal infarcts. He called the chief of surgery and invited him to come to the autopsy room and witness his dissection of the arterial supply. The chief of surgery, who probably enjoyed the challenge of intellectual combat, readily agreed. The dissection proceeded with a hushed audience as if this were a high stakes poker game. The surgeon agreed that no occlusions were present and the triumphant resident looked forward to a brilliant career.

This case was published in the New England Journal of Medicine exactly as it unfolded. It was an important contribution because it established once and for all that infarcts of the intestine occur without arterial occlusion, which was something entirely new in our understanding of pathology. The next question was the cause. It took about five years to find the answer. At first, there were studies that

---

1. Polyarteritis nodosa is a bizarre disease because inflammation of random small segments of arteries everywhere causes blood clots to form and result in multiple occlusions. This can begin with just one involved blood vessel causing a common symptom like a heart attack or a bizarre one such as gangrene of a finger. This disease is curable with treatment that suppresses the immune system, the probable source of the disease (See Appendix B). It is one of the autoimmune diseases which results from an attack on normal organs by the immune system, and which responds to the normal organ as if it were a foreign invader like a bacterial infection.

suggested that the cause was actually the treatment given for shock. Physicians administer powerful drugs, which elevate the blood pressure from the low levels of shock by causing the small systemic arteries to constrict. These small arteries normally modulate the level of blood pressure by constricting and dilating, causing the pressure to rise and fall. The suspicion was that the shock from some other cause occurred first, and that the degree and duration of arterial constriction due to the drugs was severe enough to cause infarcts as if larger arteries were occluded. This was eventually eliminated as a cause because many patients died with the same findings, but without having received these powerful drugs.

Further studies revealed one common denominator in most cases, namely, treatment with digitalis[2] for heart failure. However, the drug itself was not the cause. It became apparent that the endless variations in patterns of intestinal infarcts was due to an inability of the failing heart to maintain a sufficient propulsive force with each beat to give every organ adequate blood flow, like a useless fire hydrant without effective water pressure. Random infarcts of the intestines now made sense. A descriptive name for this disease is "the low flow syndrome."[3]

This disease was seen more and more as the numbers of octogenarians steadily rose. It was soon apparent that there was a wide spectrum of cases. Some patients had isolated infarcts of the intestines, which were easily surgically excised. Others with multiple infarcts were fatal. It also became apparent that Nature was up to its usual tactics of complicating matters in challenging ways by producing cases with both occlusive vascular disease and the low flow syndrome. Two great advances in diagnosis and therapy overcame these hurdles. One was diagnostic angiography, which enabled physicians to determine with certainty whether any arterial occlusive disease was present by injecting dye into the circulation, which

---

2. Digitalis is a powerful drug that strengthens the heart's force of contraction and relieves the symptoms of heart failure. It is also used to restore a regular heartbeat in cases prone to irregular beats. It is a classic drug in use since 1785 when it was first extracted from the plant foxglove in England by Dr. William Weathering and founded to miraculously relieve the symptoms of heart failure. Heart disease is the only indication for its use. It can be dangerous for it to be given to anyone without heart disease (See Appendix A).
3. The low flow syndrome made its appearance in the late 1950s and early 1960s when the rising numbers of octogenarians reached a critical level. This disease supervenes in patients being treated for heart failure who have lived long enough to reach the inevitable endpoint of terminal heart failure unresponsive to digitalis. The numbers of cases steadily increased over the years as life expectancy rose from 70.8 to 77.2 years from 1970 to 2001 and the percentage of all deaths of those over 85 years of age rose from 13% in 1970 to 27% in 2000.

vividly demonstrated the arterial blood supply to any organ on X-rays. This eliminated the need for an autopsy dissection to determine if there were arterial occlusions, and provided anatomical details that enabled intelligent surgical management. The other great advance was in the treatment of heart failure, which was revolutionized by the introduction of drugs called ACE-inhibitors and beta-blockers among others. These drugs clearly prolonged patients' lives way beyond the endpoint of the effectiveness of digitalis. It is still not known exactly how these drugs work. The story is not over because rising life expectancy has never leveled off.

13

A Hopeless Case with a Happy Ending

One day, one of my surgeon friends visited me. I enjoyed seeing him because he was relaxed in a contagious way that made me relax. He was a typical Midwesterner, having the gift of making you feel that he was pouring molasses over your head. He said he had a patient that I simply had to see for myself. This was a memorable event because I can recall only one other time that a surgeon invited me to see a patient. I often went to see patient's charts in medical cases with puzzling biopsies. I would encounter my friends, the doctors, at the nurses' stations, who would enjoy teasing me with comments such as "What are you doing here? Did someone die? You must be lost." As we approached the bed, I saw a quiet woman in her mid-fifties sitting up in bed, draped in a loose hospital gown and staring at me with a bland expression. She had gray hair and was moderately overweight. I noticed immediately that her yellow skin indicated jaundice. The surgeon introduced me to her and informed me that she was a farmer's wife. He then asked her if I could examine her breasts. She readily agreed and easily took her arms out of the sleeves and let the gown fall exposing her breasts.

As I looked at her breasts, I saw one of the most bizarre injuries I had ever seen. I glanced at the surgeon who responded with a sympathetic nod. What I saw was that the nipples and surrounding skin of both large pendulous breasts were completely destroyed resulting in two huge round craters. The beds of the craters were grayish-pink in color with small points of bleeding. The thought immediately struck me that I was looking at cancers that had begun in the nipple regions of both breasts and then spread out to form these terrible injuries. The surgeon then asked the patient to lie back for an abdominal examination. He gently felt the abdomen, which elicited no pain. When I examined the lower abdomen, I could feel a huge mass in her pelvis at least the size of a large grapefruit. The story that materialized in my mind was that this unfortunate woman had cancer of both breasts, which had spread to the liver causing yellow jaundice, and to the pelvic organs forming a huge mass.

We needed a biopsy to study under the microscope for a conclusive diagnosis. Therefore, with the patient's permission, the surgeon removed small amounts of tissue, from each crater of the breasts. The patient felt no pain when the biopsies were taken because the tumor contained no active nerve fibers. During this entire procedure, the patient's behavior was one of complete detachment, as if she was an impassive spectator of the proceedings. He covered the sites with loose dressings, and we left the patient's room.

We both felt that the patient had hopeless breast cancers with spread to other organs. I was fascinated by the patient's totally unemotional behavior during our visit, and then I found out that she was a farmer's wife from the boondocks of Missouri. These families learn to cope with all sorts of health problems because their individual chores are extremely essential to life on a rural farm. Only a completely disabling problem will justify time lost for a visit to the nearest physician. This patient was an example of the far advanced bizarre tumors that may develop before they seek medical help.

The following day the slides were ready for examination. I anticipated seeing a very mean variety of breast cancer. I quickly realized that this was no ordinary lesion. It did look very busy and disorganized the way cancers do but it had unique features that took awhile to register. One was that the individual cells did not look cancerous. The other became progressively clearer, that the tumor was made up of two distinct kinds of cells that looked completely benign. I had never heard of such a tumor. It looked so unique that I had to look for the illustrations of it in our major reference book for breast tumors, an Atlas of Tumors of the Breast by Dr. Fred Stewart published by the Armed Forces Institute of Pathology in Washington, DC.

I searched the reference and was delighted to find an example of this case. It turned out to be a benign tumor arising in the large ducts that deliver milk to the nipple. The bleeding nipple is characteristic of this condition, but is also a sign of breast cancer. Ordinarily, this symptom would lead most women to seek early medical attention, but not this farmer's wife. She actually was forced to seek medical attention, because the constant changes of bloodstained bandages and clothing prevented her from doing her daily physical chores. Although this is a benign tumor, it can locally destroy the nipple and surrounding skin and breast. This case illustrated how a destructive tumor can be so extensive as to suggest a cancer and yet be benign.

Upon learning that the breast lesions were benign, the surgeon then pursued the cause of the yellow jaundice. X-rays showed that she had gallstones, which obstructed the bile duct and blocked the delivery of bile from the liver to the intestine. This was a problem that could wait for a few days for surgical correction. The surgeon first removed the tumors of both breasts taking just enough surrounding normal tissues to assure that none of the tumor remained. The pendulous appearance of the breasts was improved cosmetically although the nipples were gone. Several days later he removed the gall bladder and relieved the obstruction of the bile duct.

The next challenge was the large pelvic tumor, which was diagnosed as a uterine tumor. These tumors are very common and usually benign, but occasional malignant types occur. Therefore, it is necessary to surgically remove the uterus with its tumor for microscopic study. Ultimately, the uterus was removed and contained a benign tumor the size of a cantaloupe. The patient left the hospital smelling like a rose and several pounds lighter.

14

No Help from the Best and Brightest

A routine chest X-ray showed a tumor in the chest of a man in his fifties that proved to be enlarged lymph nodes. These are sometimes called "glands" like the ones that enlarge and become palpable on the sides of the neck in children with sore throats. These organs of the immune system[1] are widely distributed throughout the body and protect us from infections by various microorganisms including viruses, bacteria, and parasites. Active infections cause them to swell and to become large enough to appear as abnormal shadows in X-rays and to be easily felt when they are close to the skin surface. Lymph nodes also can develop a distinct group of cancers, which are called "lymphomas." Enlarged lymph nodes without signs of active infection are suspicious of lymphomas. The only way to determine whether an enlarged lymph node is a lymphoma or is actively responding to a hidden infection is by microscopic examination. The patient had no complaints such as fever, pain, or weakness, and this was possible with either a hidden infection or a lymphoma. A biopsy was needed to get a definitive answer. A surgeon exposed the tumor, which revealed that it was a mass of a few enlarged lymph nodes. He excised one of them about the size of a walnut for pathologic analysis. A small sample of the specimen was taken for examination in our microbiology laboratory to see if microorganisms could be demonstrated. The rest was examined microscopically to determine whether this was an obvious lymphoma or a benign inflammatory response. I soon realized that this was a diagnostic problem because it had features of both possibilities. The problem was that some early lymphomas could masquerade as inflammatory changes, which were present. There was also some distortion of the normal structure of the node, which could mean an early lymphoma. I followed a classical rule in diagnostic pathology, which is never to make a diagnosis of cancer if there is any doubt. Since this case was one of the dreaded examples of cases that are shades

---

1. See Appendix B.

of gray between cancer and benign inflammation, I recorded my diagnosis as inflammatory.

Since I was uncertain about my diagnosis, I asked the responsible physician not to do anything until I sent off microscopic slides for consultation to three leaders in our specialty. Two of the pathologists were heads of surgical pathology in their respective university medical centers. The third headed the surgical pathology department of a large private clinic and probably saw more cases than either one of the others. One of the first two responded quickly and thought it was a lymphoma. I contacted the second pathologist by telephone to get his opinion. He sarcastically commented that anyone who considered this a lymphoma should get more training as a resident in pathology. I was pleased to hear this but felt obliged to reveal the identity of the first pathologist, who was his well-known colleague. The third pathologist called it an inflammatory response.

Two weeks went by and I received a formal report from the second pathologist, who changed his diagnosis from inflammatory response to lymphoma. This was surprising in view of his earlier arrogant response. The patient's wise physician, confronted by all this controversy, elected to do nothing and follow the patient's progress. This decision was based on the knowledge that suspicious enlarged lymph nodes showing inflammatory changes will eventually shrink if the possible cause of the inflammation is an obscure undetected virus of some sort. I eventually left St. Louis, and returned about ten years later to attend a medical meeting and visited old friends at the Jewish Hospital of Saint Louis. I ran into the doctor who was caring for this puzzling patient, and I inquired about the outcome. He responded with a gratifying smile that the lymph nodes got smaller without treatment and that the patient was doing fine.

I had kept a microscopic slide of this unusual case in my collection of problem cases with uncertain diagnoses. Years later I showed it to a colleague with whom I had trained in pathology at Montefiore Hospital many years before. He had become head of surgical pathology at the Memorial Hospital in New York and was an authority on lymph node diseases. After he inspected the slide, he looked up from his microscope and told me, "It looks like it is breaking down into a lymphoma," and he pointed out the loss of some of the lymph node's normal structure.

Who was right? I am still baffled about the diagnosis in this patient after more than forty years. The answer may always remain unknown because the failure for the lesion to progress to a lymphoma does not necessarily rule out a lymphoma. Some cancers may spontaneously regress without treatment, and some lymphomas may take years to suddenly grow forth and become obvious.

There was no right or wrong answer for this case, and perhaps the best early answer was "I don't know," but this is of no help to the doctor or patient. Therefore, pathologists do their best to arrive at their best judgment, but sometimes must admit that they simply do not know. This then requires presenting choices to the patient with a favored recommendation that the patient may or may not follow.

The good news is that advances in molecular pathology and genetics over the past twenty-five years have enabled an accurate distinction between early lymphomas and benign inflammatory changes. The advances make it possible to microscopically identify scattered cancer cells with a chemical test in a crowd of mostly benign look-alike cells. I cannot help but ponder the current need for such a test to identify terrorists. But uncertainty still persists about other diagnostic problems waiting to be eliminated by new knowledge and technology.

15

Two Deceptive Breast Tumors

It was 1960, and I had been at the Jewish Hospital of Saint Louis for about three years. My credibility as a diagnostic pathologist seemed to be established, although I sensed that every problem case became a litmus test, scrutinized by my clinical colleagues. I frequently received biopsies of breast tumors occurring in wives, sisters, and friends of the medical staff and hospital community. This was unnerving at first because I dreaded bringing the bad news of a cancer to a colleague whose sister or wife was the patient. Of course, this was very rare at Montefiore Hospital in New York City where nearly all patients were unrelated to anyone in the hospital community.

This patient was one of three sisters of a woman who was a popular administrator in the hospital and a friend to everyone including me. The patient, in her late thirties, had a breast tumor and was the only unmarried one of the sisters. When I was called to the operating room to receive the complete tumor, the surgeon assured me that the lesion was a lipoma, a benign tumor made of normal fat.

I performed a routine careful examination of the tumor, which was shaped like an intact small egg. After cutting it up into thin slices, I came across a small, hard mass less than ¼ inch in diameter buried in the fat like a small pebble. I cut through it and exposed a small, gray tumor with an irregular outline, and ray-like extensions into the surrounding yellow fat. It was hard to accept that these were the typical signs of a cancer of the breast. I proceeded with a frozen section to examine its microscopic appearance and it was unmistakably diagnostic of a cancer.

I was stunned and immediately informed the surgeon, who never realized this little cancer was in the specimen. He was also bewildered and challenged the diagnosis. I had to firmly assure him that this was a conclusive finding. He consequently proceeded to do a radical removal of the involved breast and told me that her sisters were all in the visitors' waiting room and asked if I could go tell them the bad news. I was reluctant to carry out this painful chore, but did so because it was a mandated responsibility delegated to me by the surgeon, which I could not refuse. There followed a scene of three women sobbing uncontrollably, which reminded me of childhood experiences of deaths in my family. I reassured them as best as I could by telling them that the small size of the tumor was an important indicator of a cure. I did not say anything about the other indicator, which was whether the tumor had spread to local lymph nodes, the glands of the immune system. This required a meticulous dissection and microscopic study of the lymph nodes in the axillary tissues included in the radical mastectomy specimen. The answer would be known the following day.

We applied an experimental technique, which reveals all the lymph nodes in the fatty tissue as ivory white nodules. This enables a more thorough sampling of these nodes, which can be as small as a pinhead. We found seventy-two nodes free of cancerous spread. This was good news insofar as usually fewer than forty lymph nodes are found. This reassured a favorable outcome.

A study was conducted years later, which revealed that the more thorough technique that we used actually provided no more accurate information than the standard procedure, which would have been less time consuming. It is sad to note that she died due to spread of the cancer four years later, in spite of the better outlook suggested by the small size of the tumor and absence of involved lymph nodes. This was in the days before chemotherapy of breast cancer became available. This patient was an example of what sometimes makes the choice of treatment so difficult for a breast cancer to this day.

Breast tumors often present unusual diagnostic problems as compared to tumors from other organs. The good news is that most of them in the end prove to be benign.

An example was a woman who was admitted for an excision and biopsy of a breast tumor. She was in her forties and happened to be the wife of a member of our Board of Trustees, whom I deeply respected. The board members were the most impressive people I had ever met. Aside from their wealth, they were very intelligent, clear thinking, friendly, utterly honest, and dedicated to always doing what was right.

The surgeon's pre-operative diagnosis was a benign tumor because it was discrete, firm, round and freely movable. Subsequently, he completely excised it and submitted it to me for a frozen section. It was a well-circumscribed firm tumor, which on cutting revealed a homogeneous benign looking gray-pink tumor similar to a common benign tumor of younger women called a fibroadenoma[1]. To my dismay, the frozen section revealed no fibroadenoma, but rather a tumor that looked much more complicated and could possibly be malignant. It was impossible for me to decide whether the tumor was benign or malignant on a frozen section. I needed to look at permanent sections, which are technically of better quality than frozen sections. This meant that the final answer had to be delayed until the following day, when permanent sections would be made. I informed the surgeon of the diagnostic problem, which he knew was due to limitations of frozen section technique, and he readily accepted the need for the delay. This was always a troubling event because it meant another day of anxious waiting by the patient and her family, as well as by the medical and nursing staff.

I was delighted the following day to find that the tumor was an example of sclerosing adenosis, an uncommon tumor as benign as a fibroadenoma. This tumor had microscopic features of a cancer, but its orderly growth pattern without evidence of infiltration into surrounding fat established its benign outlook. I immediately called the surgeon with the good news and issued a final report the same day. Several days later, after the patient had been reassured and gone home, her brother, a popular internist on our staff about my age, visited me. He asked me to please send the slides for consultation to a friend of his who was a nationally known pathologist and was interested in this uncommon tumor. I immediately realized that he wanted to be absolutely sure that I wasn't missing a true cancer. Having been trained myself to be skeptical and trust no one, I sympathized completely with his request, which I was also ethically bound to satisfy.

This renowned consultant trained one of my young associates, whom I sent to visit him with the microscopic slides of this case, and thought no more about it. One of the most shocking experiences of my life followed when I learned that the consultant considered it malignant. This diagnosis was not acceptable to me, because this type of tumor was very well illustrated in a definitive reference on breast tumors. This case was so typical that it could have served as good an example of its features as the case illustrated in the reference.

The reference was written by Dr. Fred Stewart, who headed the pathology department at the Memorial Sloan-Kettering Cancer Center in New York City, one of the two or three giants in surgical pathology of those days. I immediately sent the slides to Dr. Stewart for consultation. When I called him after waiting several anxious days, I cannot forget his exact opening words discussing the diagnosis: "If this were my sister, I certainly would not call it a cancer." His diagnosis was also a benign sclerosing adenosis.

---

1. The fibroadenoma is a common tumor of younger women and is benign. Pathologists love this tumor because it is so easy to diagnose on frozen section and is good news for everyone concerned, especially the patient.

About a week later the surgeon visited me. He was a typical Missourian, of the ilk of Harry Truman. He told me that in the attempt to end this confusion, he visited the consultant, who he knew very well, and questioned him about his diagnosis. He related that the consultant had seen an article about this tumor in a British medical journal, which described features of early malignant change, which he noticed in this case. Now we know that a rare case of sclerosing adenosis may become malignant, but when it does, the cancerous changes are not subtle, but full-blown and easily recognized. Ten years later, I ran into the patient's brother at a national medical conference and asked him how she was doing. He said that there were no more problems with the breast tumor.

16

A Deadly New Life Form

An elderly woman in her seventies was admitted to the hospital in the late 1950s for terminal care by one of our young neurologists. She had an undiagnosed disease of the nervous system. The illness began less than a year before her admission. The first symptom was blurring of vision of both eyes, which got progressively worse. An eye specialist examined her and found that the eyes were perfectly normal. The mirror of our surroundings in the eyes, called the retina, was intact. This meant that there was an injury that interrupted nerve signals somewhere between the retinas in the eyeballs and the visual centers in the gray matter[1] of the brain, where "seeing" actually occurs. The injury could be anywhere in this pathway including the terminal visual centers.

As the loss of vision progressed, the neurologist was able to localize the injury in the gray matter of the brain including the visual centers. The major clue for

---

1. The gray matter is another name for the cerebral cortex, the outer layer surrounding the brain, where all of our senses are registered for us to experience. It is also the source of all of our bodily functions like physical activity, speech, memory, intelligence and the miracle of creative abilities. The centers that control all of our organs, over which we have no conscious control as we do in the use of our hands or any physical activity, are also represented in the gray matter. These include the involuntary activities of the cardiovascular, gastrointestinal and urinary systems. The cerebral cortex is one huge database with built-in software that is mostly independent of our will, but which can think and create new software. The visual centers are where we actually "see" our surroundings. There is a neat nervous network in the brain between the eyes and the visual centers on the surface of the back of the brain. The retinas are lined by layers of highly specialized nerve cells, which are individually activated by shades of light and colors. The countless impulses travel through the network and a single major relay in the brain to reach the visual centers. Here, the impulses stimulate special nerve cells that result in the images we see. I am reminded of the countless impulses in an e-mail, which can similarly transmit a color image appearing on the monitor screen, which amounts to a man-made visual center.

this was the progressive dementia with loss of memory and intelligence that ensued, which occurs with many diseases involving gray matter including the most common one, Alzheimer's disease. Progressive dementia is typical of a degenerative disease of the cerebral cortex. As loss of vision progressed, bizarre behavior and speech ensued, which also results from any gray matter disease. She became totally blind and unaware of time, place and her identity. She slipped into coma and died several days later from aspiration pneumonia[2].

The clinical diagnosis was "degenerative disease of the central nervous system," which simply means that there is a destructive disease of the cerebral cortex that causes severe dementia. A specific disease cannot be diagnosed because many different diseases of unknown cause produce this terminal condition. The only way to identify the disease is by microscopic study of the gray matter in a biopsy taken during life or at autopsy.

Many diseases can cause progressive dementia, including Alzheimer's disease, but which do not cause complete blindness. I spoke to the neurologist to try and get his best guess about the possible diagnosis before the autopsy. He could not make an intelligent suggestion, which was not surprising because of the limited knowledge and rarity of these diseases. You can fill a textbook of neuropathology with all the possible diseases that can cause cerebral cortical disease, including infectious, neoplastic, and cardiovascular diseases. The degenerative diseases of the nervous system are so named because their causes are unknown and can also fill a textbook of neuropathology. Aside from the more common diseases such as Alzheimer's disease, multiple sclerosis and Lou Gehrig's disease, there are many other very rare types. It was for this reason that I began this autopsy feeling overwhelmed and wondering whether I would be able to nail down a definite diagnosis.

The general autopsy findings were normal except for the aspiration pneumonia. The exposed brain looked deceptively normal. I had no idea what to expect to find in the microscopic studies. I followed a routine system of studying tissues from designated parts of the brain, including the visual centers. The microscopic findings relieved my anxieties. There was a severe degree of destruction of the gray matter characteristic of a very rare disease named after the German neuropathologists who first described it, Creutzfeld-Jakob disease (CJD). This one

---

2. Coma may cause loss of the normal reflex to cough up anything that gets into the airways and into the lungs, such as foods and liquids. We habitually constantly swallow saliva without conscious effort. The loss of the ability to swallow in coma results in aspiration of saliva into the lungs. Saliva is loaded with oral bacteria, which cause aspiration pneumonia. Antibiotics have no effect on the infection because of the continuous influx of contaminated saliva.

looked the same as a single case I saw at Montefiore Hospital in my training days. Her story of the disease was typical of one known variant, which begins with progressive loss of vision. I recall my encounter with the young neurologist when I told him about my findings. He reacted as one who had never before seen a case and was surprised to have encountered such an extremely rare disease.

The story does not end here because of surprising and sometimes bizarre later developments in Creutzfeldt-Jacob disease (CJD). Investigators thought that CJD might be a chronic viral disease because of a known disease of the nervous system of sheep called scrapie, which caused similar microscopic changes in the brain. Scrapie was deliberately transmitted from diseased to healthy sheep to determine whether it was due to an infectious agent. Indeed it was transmissible, but the incubation period took from months to years before symptoms appeared and the causative agent was never identified. This long delay in the onset of symptoms led to the concept of the "slow virus diseases," assuming that the cause was an unusual but "slow" unknown virus.

A fatal disease of the nervous system in New Guinea natives called kuru was known to look like CJD microscopically and was also regarded as a slow virus disease. Its infectiousness was proven by transmission to chimpanzees. Painstaking investigations in the late 1950s led to the discovery that the pathway of transmission among natives was their ritual of eating the brains of the dead in all their burial ceremonies. Natives who ate the brains of victims of kuru acquired the disease. Ending this cannibalistic practice greatly reduced the numbers of diseased natives. A Nobel Prize for this solution was awarded to D. Carleton Gajdusek of the National Institutes of Health in 1976. This was worth a Nobel Prize because he demonstrated an entirely new way that an infectious disease could be transmitted.

I was then startled to learn in the late 1970s that too many recipients of corneal transplants[3] acquired CJD, considering its extreme rarity. It turned out that the donors of these transplants were autopsied cases whose eyes were donated to eye surgeons to obtain the corneas for transplants into living patients with diseased corneas causing blindness. All the donors had died of CJD, which at the time was regarded as a fatal cerebral degenerative disease of unknown cause. This publicized development left no doubt among physicians that CJD was indeed an infectious disease.

---

3. The cornea is the thin translucent layer of tissue on the surface of the eye over the pupils. Various diseases can cause scarring of the cornea making it opaque and causing blindness, which can be eliminated by simply cutting off the diseased cornea and replacing it with a normal cornea from a deceased donor. This was the first example of an organ transplant from one person to another.

More bizarre examples of the infectious transmissibility of CJD appeared.

Other new cases had undergone diagnostic studies to plan treatments for epilepsy. These studies included taking readings of the electrical activity of the brain during surgery with metallic electrodes that contacted the surface of the brain. It turned out that the electrodes had been previously used on cases with eventually proven CJD. It became clear that the method used to chemically sterilize these delicate electrodes between cases had no effect on the infectious agent causing the disease. The electrodes were infectious once they had been applied to an early case whose major symptom was the onset of epilepsy. The failure of the sterilization procedure to kill the infectious agent was totally unexpected and another frightening characteristic of the deadly agent.

A tragic example of a means of transmission of CJD was the virtual epidemic in the late 1980s among adults thirty to fifty years of age, who all had one common source of infection. They were all dwarfs in early childhood and were given injections of pituitary growth hormone[4] to enable normal growth. The only source of the human growth hormone was the human pituitary gland obtained from autopsies. The growth hormone from other animal species was useless because the human immune system reacted to them as foreign material and neutralized their activity. The supply of glands from autopsies was less than the ideal number needed for the treatment of all dwarfs. This shortage led to the need for a National Pituitary Foundation, which was set up at Johns Hopkins University to pool all of the pituitary glands gathered from the autopsy services of all hospitals in the United States. They combined batches of glands from which the precious hormone was extracted and distributed evenhandedly to pediatricians in the United States. The supply was never optimal but effective in minimizing dwarfism. The reason for the high numbers of victims was the batching of pituitary glands together for processing in the preparation of extract. A batch contaminated by one gland from a case of CJD could conceivably infect dozens of recipients. This experience highlighted two frightening characteristics of the infectious agent. One was another demonstration of the resistance of the agent to usual chemical methods of sterilization. The other was the long incubation period of thirty to forty years for the disease to become manifest after infection in childhood.

---

4. The pituitary gland is the source of growth hormone, which is one of many hormones the gland secretes that affects growth and the secretion of hormones from other endocrine glands such as the thyroid, adrenal glands and sex organs. It is called the master gland because of its universal control of other glands and is well protected in the floor of the skull beneath the brain.

Advances in genetic engineering have eliminated the need for human pituitary glands as the only source of pure human growth hormone, which is a protein[5]. It is now possible to modify the DNA[6] of bacteria to produce a pure supply of any selected single protein by implanting in them the single human gene with the accurate blueprint. Today, bacteria that have been modified by the addition of the human gene for growth hormone produce adequate amounts of the pure hormone to treat dwarfs.

The most recent outbreak in the early 1990s of a disease like CJD was mad cow disease in Great Britain. Human beings acquired the disease by eating beef products contaminated by slaughtered cows having the disease. This again demonstrated the great risk of infection because established methods of sterilization and cooking beef did not kill the agent. There have also been rare incidents of infections among those in contact with diseased nervous system tissues, including neurosurgeons, pathologists and technologists.

The demonstration that CJD was without question an infectious disease was its transmission to chimpanzees in the late 1960s. This then stimulated investigators to discover the infectious agent and learn as much as possible about its structure with a view to rapid diagnosis, possible treatments, and prevention. This required animals such as mice and hamsters to be experimentally infected from human cases. It was a monumental task because of the long incubation period taking up to a year before infected animals could be studied. This compares to incubation periods of a few days in usual bacterial and viral infectious diseases. The leader in this research was Stanley B. Prusiner, who devoted more than twenty years to the goals of isolating the agent, determining its structure, and how it multiplies in the victim. His fruitful efforts astounded the scientific com-

---

5. The bulk of our tissues and most hormones are proteins, which is why meat is the richest source of proteins in our diet. The basic protein particle is a large molecule made up of a long chain of smaller molecules called amino acids. There are 17 types of amino acids, which are arranged in chains of numbers of types and sequences unique to each of the some 30,000 proteins, of which we are made.
6. DNA (deoxyribonucleic acid). DNA is the major component of genes in our cells. These are huge molecules made up of long chains of larger complex molecules called nucleic acids. There are only four types of nucleic acids, but their different arrangements in types and numbers are unique for each of some 30,000 genes in our cells. It is no coincidence that the numbers of genes and proteins are equivalent, because it is the DNA in genes that provides cells with the blueprints and materials for the assembling of each of the individual proteins. The DNA also provides the scaffolding for the production of its own duplicates in the two new cells resulting from the division of a parent cell. This is its key role in the reproduction of all living things.

munity because of revelations that opened a whole new chapter in knowledge about infectious disease. It is no exaggeration to say that his discoveries were as important as the discovery of viruses when Martinus Willem Beijerinck (1851–1931) found that diseased plants contain bacteria-free fluids, which infected other plants. He called the agent a *virus*, a Latin word, which means "poison." It took thirty-seven more years in 1935 for Wendell M. Stanley to demonstrate that the virus causing a disease of tobacco plants was actually a living particle containing protein. Prusiner's research not only led to the discovery of a whole new type of infectious agent, but also to a new type of living matter unlike all known plant and animal life.

Prusiner eventually succeeded in isolating enough of the infectious agent to determine its molecular structure. The isolation alone took years and was a major advance. The analysis of its structure revealed that it was simply another protein with no DNA. This was the first shocker because all living things are made up of proteins and DNA. One must understand the relationship between proteins and DNA to realize that no scientist would have ever dreamed of living matter lacking DNA. This is because DNA has always been essential to the multiplication of all living things and is the blueprint for the manufacture of some 30,000 different proteins. The immediate question that arose once the agent proved to be a simple protein was how it multiplied like any infectious agent. No one ever dreamed of any form of reproduction that did not involve DNA. More surprises followed.

The analysis of this protein, including the kinds, number, and arrangements of several hundred amino acids composing it, led to a startling discovery. It turned out that a protein identical to the CJD agent was a normal component of our tissues, but with one difference. The three dimensional arrangement of the amino acid chains was different from the CJD agent. In a nutshell, its twists in the loops of chains of amino acids were different. It is well known by biochemists that two molecules made up of the identical sequence and types of units but with different spatial shapes can have remarkably different chemical properties. Exactly how the CJD protein multiplies is unknown and worth a Nobel Prize, but it is thought that once it gets into any tissue as the seed of a demon, it somehow causes the victim's normal corresponding protein to change to the same deadly configuration. It is thought that it may not multiply to produce copies of itself in addition to its normal counterparts in cells, but by causing its normal counterparts to change their spatial shape to the deadly form with a continuing domino effect. I am reminded of science fiction themes where aliens from outer space come here and convert humans to copies of their own kind. Somehow, this agent targets the nervous system and kills nerve cells. It is puzzling that it can be found in other organs that it does not injure.

Dr. Stanley B. Prusiner received the Nobel Prize in 1997 for his unraveling of the structure of the CJD agent and its amazing features. He coined the name "prion" for this new form of infectious agent from the descriptive name "protein infectious agent." This was a monumental discovery for a number of reasons. There are now possibilities of early diagnosis, treatment and prevention of CJD. Today, the only way to establish a diagnosis of CJD is by a brain biopsy or at autopsy. The knowledge of the exact chemistry of the CJD protein makes it possible to design a blood laboratory test for rapid diagnosis. Its structure is also the key to designing drugs that can block the deadly protein from converting a normal type to a copy of itself. The fact that the CJD protein structure is stable makes it an ideal subject for a vaccine that can be chemically designed to induce the immune system to inactivate it whenever it may appear.

There are other exciting possibilities. We had four million cases of Alzheimer's disease and one million cases of Parkinson's disease compared to four hundred cases of CJD in 2000. Both of these diseases and many other diseases of unknown cause of the nervous system produce abnormal proteins but they are not infectious. Since the hallmark of each is a diagnostic unique protein, a mechanism similar to CJD may account for the onset of these diseases. Consider any protein in any organ undergoing a spatial change of some sort that becomes injurious and recruits others to the same deadly form. The diseases of unknown cause fill more than half of the pages in medical textbooks. It would be surprising if CJD turned out to be the only example of a prion disease. All these possibilities are now under investigation. The importance of Prusiner's contribution cannot be overstated.

The recognition of this infectious agent led to the introduction of strict procedures to protect pathologists and their assistants from infection. The most effective disinfectants are Chlorox and formic acid. The only way to guarantee them protection is to stop doing autopsies. I have since been involved with one other case diagnosed during life. Autopsies on such cases are imperative to determine for a fact whether a fatal disease is CJD disease by microscopic study. What we don't know can hurt us.

1966–73, Montefiore Hospital, New York City, Attending Pathologist

17

The Mother of All Cancers

It was 1968, and this 78-year-old woman, who was being treated for coronary artery disease, was sitting in her physician's waiting room for a routine follow-up visit. She was doing well after responding to treatment for angina pectoris, a characteristic chest pain caused by exertion and relieved by rest. Suddenly, she shocked other waiting patients by literally toppling over to the floor and dying without making a sound.

The family granted an autopsy. The most probable cause of such a sudden death was ventricular fibrillation[1]. The resident pathologist, who was assigned to this autopsy expected to find severe coronary arteriosclerosis, the most common cause of sudden death. When he made routine surgical incisions into the chest cavity to expose the heart, he was startled by a massive hemorrhage of about a half gallon of blood, which filled the left chest cavity and compressed the left lung. This amounted to more than half of the total blood volume in the body. The resident had never experienced such a surprise and called me to help him find the source and cause of the hemorrhage.

When I was called for consultation, I was shocked as much as the resident, because I had never seen this myself, but I knew of possibilities to consider and investigate. The first task was to get all of the blood out in order to find the source. I guided the resident to do this carefully without complicating matters by a careless dissection producing false sources of hemorrhage.

The surface of the lung itself was carefully examined for a source of hemorrhage without success. Attention was then directed to the inner surface of the chest cavity, the large space around the lung. We were surprised to find that there

---

1. Ventricular fibrillation is a sudden loss of steady heartbeats replaced by a completely ineffective trembling heart, with a sudden loss of circulating blood. The effect is the same as when normal heartbeats stop and is instantly fatal. This grossly abnormal heart rhythm can occur in heart diseases of all kinds and is most often seen with coronary artery disease.

was a small hole about halfway down the aorta[2] measuring no more than about 3/16ths of an inch in diameter. It leaked blood and was the obvious source of hemorrhage. I was aware of only two possible causes for such a perforation, in the absence of a bullet wound or the stab wound of an ice pick. One was an infection of heart valves called bacterial endocarditis[3], which was 100% fatal in the pre-antibiotic era. I figured that this might have happened in this case, but she had no history of fever and feeling rotten as is characteristic of endocarditis.

The heart in this case was examined with great care under sterile conditions to view the possibly infected heart valves, and to obtain some of the infected tissue for a culture to identify the bacteria. We used a technique to examine the heart under sterile conditions, as in an operating room, which was the clever invention by one of our residents, Dr. Conrad Tsai from Taiwan. He conceived of a technique to enable getting uncontaminated samples of infected valves from cases dying of endocarditis. It was essential to identify the bacteria at autopsy, grow it and test it for sensitivity to antibiotics for the sake of future cases. New strains of bacteria causing endocardititis constantly appear and it is obligatory to identify them and determine the best antibiotic for cure. We used the sterile technique and carefully examined the four heart valves and found them normal and uninfected.

I was aware of only one remaining possible way that a perforation of the aorta could occur. I suggested that this could be an example of a very rare disease called polyarteritis nodosa[4]. I reassured everyone that the microscopic examination would reveal this answer but I was surprised often enough by unexpected findings

---

2. The aorta is a huge arterial trunk, as big as a garden hose, which originates from the heart and supplies blood to the entire body. It passes down through the chest in front of the spine roughly in the midline to supply the chest, abdomen, pelvis and legs. One can see the left side of the aorta as a linear bulge through the translucent membrane lining the left chest cavity, as it passes downward to supply all the organs and lower half of the body.
3. Bacterial endocarditis is a growth of infectious bacteria, which occurs on the heart valve with tissue destruction, blood clot formation and severe inflammation. The combination of the bacterial growth and clot formation results in an irregular friable mass covering the valve like a fungus called a vegetation. Bits of it can break off and be carried in the bloodstream. These infected bits can obstruct small arteries elsewhere and cause infected infarcts. It can be a devastating disease. One of its characteristic complications is the lodging of a small and infected particle in the mouth of a small artery branching off the aorta. It then continues to fester and destroy tissue. Eventually, the aortic wall is focally destroyed and perforates, which is fatal with massive hemorrhage, as in this case.

to be prepared for anything. I impatiently waited for the microscopic slides, which would be ready the next day.

We were amazed to find that the margin of the hole in the aortic wall was made up of highly malignant cancer cells, which were huge with bizarre microscopic features. It was impossible to tell whether the cancer arose from one of the organs in the chest or abdomen, or from one of the several connective tissues of the body like fibrous, fat or muscle tissue. Cancers usually bear some resemblance to the tissue of origin. However, some appear so bizarre microscopically that it is impossible to suggest an organ source of origin. Such a cancer is called an "undifferentiated malignant tumor." Cancer cells had apparently spread in the bloodstream and lodged in a small blood vessel in the wall of the aorta and continued to multiply there. The proliferating cells occupied the space remaining from the destruction of aortic wall cells until a full thickness of the aortic wall was focally made up purely of cancerous cells. These cancerous growths have no tensile strength like a normal aortic wall. The cells were simply blown away under arterial pressure like a cork out of a champagne bottle, leaving behind a hole lined by remaining cancer cells.

The remainder of the autopsy did reveal a small globular tumor deep in the thyroid gland, which was not seen until a cut was made into the gland. It measured about ½ inch in diameter and no more was thought about it until it was studied under the microscope as a routine procedure. Small benign nodular thyroid tumors are found frequently at autopsy. The lesion proved to be a highly malignant tumor of the thyroid gland, which is uncommon but well known. It bears no resemblance to thyroid tissue, being completely undifferentiated, and typically occurs in the elderly over age 70. One popular name for it is "giant cell carcinoma of the thyroid gland." There are a few cancers that are among the most malignant and this is one of them. No one has ever been cured of this tumor by surgical excision, because it spreads in the bloodstream so early. Survival is for a few months at most. I was destined to see one more case several years later at the Mount Sinai Hospital in Hartford, Connecticut that first showed up as a shower of small nodules under the skin. There was no obvious tumor of the thyroid gland on physical examination. A biopsy of one nodule looked the same as this case and the source in the thyroid gland was confirmed.

---

4. Polyarteritis nodosa is a disease of arteries that produces random scattered foci of destruction of arterial walls with intense inflammation and occasional fatal ruptures. The cause is unknown but it is thought to be one of the autoimmune diseases, which are due to an attack by the immune system on normal organs as if they were foreign organisms such as bacteria (see Appendix B).

18

A Stroke That Wasn't a Stroke

An 82-year-old retired schoolteacher suddenly developed a typical stroke with sudden loss of consciousness. He was revived in a short time and, while his speech was intact, he was disoriented and confused, and was unable to move the paralyzed left arm and leg. Although he was a heavy smoker, he had enjoyed relatively good health without hypertension, diabetes or heart disease. He did suffer from emphysema, but was not disabled by it. A typical stroke usually improves over two to three weeks, with return of normal mental faculties, and, often, with clearing of the paralysis. One has to understand the characteristics of a stroke in order to know how recovery occurs. The most common cause is the sudden deprivation of the blood supply to a part of the brain in the vicinity of the nerve tracts that enable all voluntary muscular activities including speech. The loss of blood supply is due to narrowing or occlusion of arteries by arteriosclerosis. The resulting injury is death of the region deprived of a blood supply, known as an infarct. A similar problem can occur in a typical heart attack, called a myocardial infarct.

The brain differs from all other organs insofar as healthy brain tissue surrounding any sort of injury, such as an infarct, undergoes a reaction that is not seen in other organs. The reaction is called cerebral swelling. Body fluids pour into the intercellular spaces between healthy nerve cells and their nerve tracts swelling the region surrounding the infarct. The least volume of swollen brain tissue surrounding a pea-sized infarct may be that of a peach as compared to a pea. The soaking of brain matter by accumulating body water knocks out all normal nervous activity. For example, swelling of a region that includes the passage of nerve tracts, which transmit signals to move muscles or feel pain, touch and temperature, causes paralysis and loss of sensation of the affected side of the body. The early temporary swelling results in a much greater loss of nervous function than those due to the irreversible destruction of the actual infarct. Indeed, all lost functions may return because there are many silent parts of the brain where an infarct may occur without permanent disabilities.

Our patient did not show any improvement after one week, but seemed stable and rested quietly. He was still being observed during the second week when he became stuporous and then comatose. He developed a pneumonia, which did not respond to antibiotics and he expired. The autopsy revealed a bronchopneumonia of the lower right lung due to coma with aspiration of saliva from the oral cavity. This is a frequent finding among some patients who have lost their cough reflex, and can occur whenever there is a persistent loss of brain activity as may occur with extensive cerebral swelling.

The unexpected finding was a cancer of the right upper lung situated on the surface next to the midline structures in the chest. These structures include the spine behind the esophagus and trachea giving off the bronchi to each lung, and the heart with all of its great arteries and veins. The problem was that the shadow of this tumor was hidden on the chest X-ray in the large midline shadow cast by all these larger structures. This was a round tumor on the lung surface about the size of a quarter and about 3/8ths of an inch thick. It invaded and was adherent to the opposing surface of the midline structures, with which it blended imperceptibly on the X-rays.

Further investigation revealed that the lesion in the brain was not an infarct but a focus of spread of the lung cancer to the brain called a metastasis. Cerebral edema occurs with any injury to the brain including infarcts, abscesses, brain tumors, and metastatic cancer. The persistence of edema in this case because of the persistence of injury due to a growing cancer was the basis for no improvement. Occasionally, the first symptom of an occult cancer may be a metastasis to the brain. The presenting symptom may be indistinguishable from a stroke due to arteriosclerosis. The stroke appears when the cerebral edema surrounding the tumor extends to involve nerve tracts with paralysis, as in this case. During the autopsy, other smaller metastases in the brain, lymph nodes, liver, kidneys, and adrenal glands were also discovered. This case illustrates how an unavoidable error may make no difference in the outcome of a hopeless fatal disease.

The CAT scan was introduced about five years later in the early 1970s. A routine study of the chest and brain would have easily suggested the correct diagnosis in this case.

19

A Cancer Can Do Anything

A 56-year-old man lost twenty pounds in weight over a period of six months due to a loss of appetite. He also became progressively weaker and had no pain. He had a thorough physical examination, which revealed no abnormalities other than the signs of weight loss. The blood chemistries were al! normal. A blood count did reveal a mild anemia. The chest X-ray showed multiple small nodular lesions varying in size from about ¼ to ¾ inches in diameter, suggesting metastatic cancer from an unknown source. The stool was negative for blood suggesting that the cancer was not somewhere in the intestines. He was admitted to the hospital when he lost consciousness one day and was found to have a pulse rate of 40, instead of a normal rate of 70 to 80. An EKG revealed an abnormal cardiac rhythm called complete heart block. This dangerously slow heart rate meant that there was some sort of injury to the nervous system of the heart itself [1].

He died three days after admission despite the appropriate management of heart block. The autopsy revealed a cancer of the pancreas located in the part

---

1. The intrinsic nervous system of the heart is called the *conduction system,* which is a natural pacemaker and generates the regular impulses that cause the heart to contract rhythmically throughout life. It is made up of two major parts. Each impulse is first generated in the first part called the *sinoatrial node.* This is a small organ the size of a melon seed, which is located in the wall of the right atrium, the chamber that first receives venous blue blood from the entire body. The impulse travels through the wall of the atrium to the second part in the wall of the ventricles. This part consists of a small trunk of specialized heart muscle the size of a grain of rice, which, like the trunk of a tree, has countless microscopic branches throughout the heart. It is called the *atrioventricular node.* The impulse from the sinoatrial node triggers an impulse from the *atrioventicular node* and its branches to both ventricles resulting in their simultaneous contractions. The familiar electrocardiogram is a recording of the impulses generated first by the sinoatrial node followed by the impulses of the atrioventricular node. Heart disease often causes abnormalities of the electrocardiogram because of injury anywhere in the conduction system.

called the tail [2]. In this case, the cancer had spread locally to lymph nodes, the glands of the immune system, as well as the liver and lungs, both of which contained similar nodular metastases. The heart also showed a few small nodular metastases.

Injury of the atrioventricular node due to disease can end its rhythmic response to impulses from the sinoatrial node. This is called complete heart block and results in a very slow heart rate down to a pulse of 40 or less, which can cause fainting or sudden death. The reason the heartbeats do not end altogether is that there is a capability of the branches of the atrioventricular node to generate regular impulses but at a slower rate that is about half the normal rate. The most common cause of this problem is arteriosclerotic heart disease. Today the solution is an artificial pacemaker about the size of a pocket watch, which is permanently placed under the skin of the upper chest. It produces impulses carried to the heart wall by a wire, which is threaded through a vein entering the heart, where it is attached to the inner surface.

We were curious to see whether a microscopic examination of the conduction system would reveal the cause of the complete heart block. We were amazed to find that cells of the cancer of the pancreas completely replaced the tiny encapsulated atrioventricular node. Its diameter was about the size of the head of a pin. He was doomed to die eventually even if the heart block did not occur, but it probably did contribute to an earlier death.

---

2. The pancreas has a characteristic shape similar to a tadpole, with a rounded head at one end blending into a longer body with a tip called the tail. Cancers of the body and tail of the pancreas are notoriously difficult to diagnose early because any eventual symptom is due to metastases to other organs. Cancers located in the head often call attention to their presence by compressing and obstructing the bile duct, which conducts bile from the liver to the intestines. The obstruction causes painless jaundice, which requires investigation for its cause (See anecdote 11).

1973–92, Mount Sinai Hospital, Hartford, Connecticut, Chief of Pathology

20

A Rare Cause of a Rare Disease

A 67-year-old man was admitted to the hospital with progressive weight loss of thirty pounds for six months due to loss of appetite. He had a history of coronary artery disease and a heart attack two years before. He was stable until one year ago, when he developed the sudden onset of shortness of breath with swelling of one leg.

The swelling was due to edema, an abnormal accumulation of water in the tissues. The edema was due to blood clots in veins blocking the return of venous blood from the leg to the lungs. The damming back of venous blood below the obstructing clots engorged the venous tributaries and capillaries forcing excess water to leak through their walls into the surrounding tissues.

The shortness of breath was due to blood clots, which ultimately broke loose from the leg veins and were carried to the lungs. A blood clot can be big enough to block venous blood flow into a significant portion of the lungs. More rapid and difficult breathing compensates for the loss of a sufficient functioning lung to oxygenate blood normally.

Diagnostic imaging and blood chemical studies were consistent with blood clots jammed into a lung. He was immediately treated with blood thinners to prevent the further formation of blood clots anywhere. These thinners work by reducing the ability of the blood to clot, with the drawback that they can cause a side effect of too great a bleeding tendency. In order to prevent bleeding complications, regular tests are done that measure how long it takes blood to clot. The tests enable doctors to control the dosage of blood thinner to prevent blood clots and also prevent bleeding complications from over dosage. He did very well and was discharged and placed on lifelong therapy with blood thinners, as is usual in some cases.

The onset of weight loss with increasing weakness was very gradual. His physician eventually saw him and immediately noted the marked wasting and pallor apparent on physical examination. He admitted the patient back to the hospital with an admission diagnosis of metastatic cancer, primary site to be determined. The diagnostic workup that was initiated included imaging studies of the skeleton, lungs, kidneys and intestines for a primary cancerous lesion. Studies were also done for evidence of chronic infection, such as tuberculosis, which could also cause weight loss. Routine screening blood counts and chemistries were also done. The patient died unexpectedly on the fifth hospital day, without an established diagnosis.

The autopsy revealed no evidence of a cancer. The heart did show the scar of a previous old heart attack. There were no blood clots in the lungs, which were not expected because of the blood-thinning treatment he was getting. Both adrenal glands[1] showed extensive old and recent bleeding, making each appear as a globular bloodstained mass measuring about 2 inches in diameter. There was extensive necrosis of the glands, and a well developed healing and scarring response to the slow persistent bleeding. This revelation suggested that the patient might have died of adrenal insufficiency, which is also known as Addison's disease[2]. Destruction of the adrenal glands causes Addison's disease, which is fatal if left untreated. The cause of death is an elevation of the blood concentration of potassium to deadly levels. This is normally prevented by cortisone, a hormone secreted by normal adrenal glands. Potassium blood levels normally modulate the rhythm of the heart. The failure of the glands to secrete sufficient cortisone results in unrestrained high blood potassium concentrations with an abrupt end of heartbeats and sudden death. It is for this reason that an intravenous infusion of potassium is used in some state prisons for executions. In recent years, a physician introduced controversial assisted suicides using potassium infusions.

The glands secrete several hormones, which have other far-reaching controls on maintenance of life affecting the heart, liver, kidneys, nervous system,

---

1. The adrenal glands are located on each side straddling the tops of the kidneys. Their normal size and shape is similar to that of a light tan Brazil nut.
2. Addison's disease is very rare and is occasionally unrecognized before death, which can occur unexpectedly and an autopsy reveals destruction of the glands. The most common cause of Addison's disease prior to the 1950s was tuberculosis, before effective anti-tubercular drugs were developed. The most common cause today is an abnormality of the immune system (See Appendix B). This disease is one example of many that are called the autoimmune diseases. The immune system reacts to adrenal cells like foreign invaders. A stampede of destructive lymphocytes and other cell types invades the glands disrupting and obscuring its normal structure like a town devastated by a tornado. The cause and molecular basis of these diseases are unknown and the subjects of major medical research.

immune system, and voluntary muscles. The hormone's effect on potassium levels is just one of many actions maintaining a normal salt and water composition of the body as a whole, including the concentrations of sodium and chlorine. Our waterproof skin confines the watery environment in which all of our tissues live. It is revealing to understand that the chemistry of our watery environment is very similar to seawater, as if our tissues live underwater like fish. The maintenance of life requires the preservation of a stable concentration of each of the elements that are dissolved in both body water and seawater.

The conclusion that death was due to Addison's disease cannot be made alone from how the glands appear in the autopsy room and under the microscope. This is because of their high functional reserve, which means that they have to be almost completely destroyed to result in measurable fatal concentrations of potassium in blood. The absence of viable adrenal tissue in microscopic studies is not absolute proof because viable microscopic foci might be seen if the entire glands were studied microscopically. That means a feat producing about 30,000 slides, which is impractical. For this reason, proof requires evidence that the blood potassium levels were fatally elevated during life, or that the concentration of cortisone in the blood was sufficiently lowered. One day prior to death, a potassium value was reported as 7 units, which could be fatal, because the normal potassium concentration is 3.5 to 5.0 units. This chemical evidence proved that Addison's disease was, indeed, the cause of death. Today, suspicion of Addison's disease would also be checked by a blood cortisone test, which was not rapidly available thirty years ago.

There was one other finding consistent with adrenal insufficiency. The measurement of the blood count includes a measure of the white cells in the blood, which are part of the immune system. There are five different kinds of white cells that are measured. One of them is called an eosinophile. Normal adrenal function prevents elevation of the normal number of these cells higher than 2 to 3 units. The eosinophile count in this case was 13 units, another indication of loss of vital adrenal function. Unfortunately, these abnormal findings were unknown by the physician, because they were reported shortly before unexpected death occurred.

Anti-coagulant therapy prevents excessive blood clotting in individuals who are prone to form clots in veins. However, there is a risk of unexpected bleeding occurring even when tests reveal an ideal degree of blood thinning. The most common manifestation is blood in the urine, which can be managed at once. An unsuspected gastric ulcer or an undiagnosed cancer can be disclosed by the onset of bleeding during treatment. There are other unusual patterns of bleeding as occurred in this patient.

The clinical behavior of Addison's disease is nonspecific. Loss of appetite with weight loss[3] could have occurred with a cancer, heart failure, a chronic infection, an autoimmune disease, or even mental depression. This case illustrates the dictum that the only scientific basis for a diagnosis of cancer is pathologic proof by biopsy or needle aspiration cytology. The syndrome in this case did suggest advanced cancer, but this was only a clinical diagnosis subject to pathologic proof, or elimination by demonstrating another cause. Addison's disease is the sort of entity one has to constantly consider in any obscure chronic debilitating syndrome, in spite of its rarity. The reason is that lifelong therapy with cortisone is curative. CAT scans and MRI studies of the adrenal glands in cases with obscure syndromes should help to result in earlier recognition of this complication.

---

3. The specific cause of weight loss in chronic debilitating disease of any cause is unknown. There is a remarkable small part of the brain called the hypothalamus, which controls appetite. It also controls all of our involuntary functions including body temperature, feeding to satiety, thirst, digestion, urination, defecation, and sexual drive. It is located at the center of the base of the brain and controls the pituitary gland, which secretes hormones controlling the activity all of the other glands that secrete hormones, including the thyroid, adrenal, testicular and ovarian glands. The hypothalamus has feeding and satiety centers, which are somehow involved with weight loss and are probably affected by any debilitating disease. The changes in the chemistry of the watery environment of all cells and the role of the immune system in chronic disease somehow depress the feeding center. There are voids in knowledge of the details of how the feeding center is normally roused and inhibited.

21

The Jogger Who Fainted

This case is an example of a patient's deceptive response to disease, which resulted in a missed lifesaving diagnosis. The syndrome presented by this patient was fainting while jogging. Fainting due to physical exertion is rare but is the classical symptom of a rare malady called primary pulmonary hypertension. This is a disease of unknown cause that occurs in young adults. It is a functional disease of the small arteries in the lungs [1].

An athletic 52-year-old insurance agent, who appeared lean and healthy, experienced a transient episode of light-headedness and blurring of vision, followed by a brief fainting spell and falling while jogging. An identical episode recurred during another jogging session, which prompted him to seek medical care. His

---

1. Normal arteries throughout the body have the capability of increasing or decreasing their calibers by contracting or relaxing the specialized muscle cells in their walls. The action is similar to making a tight fist or relaxing it. This is not under conscious control and is constantly progressing during life. Blood flow to the various organs does not occur constantly through all the small arteries. Most of them are contracted at any one time and the remaining numbers of dilated small arteries provide the blood supply needed for life support. All of the small arteries participate in rhythmic contractions and dilatations. For example, imagine that the spots on a leopard each represent a dilated cluster of small arteries and the skin between having the contracted small arteries. The image of a leopard with constantly shifting spots would be an ideal illustration of how the blood supply to an organ is actually distributed and always changing.

    It has been estimated that if all the small arteries in the lungs dilated at once, the entire blood volume would pool in the lungs, resulting in sudden death. Apparently, the numbers of small arteries in the lungs contracting at any one time is far greater than normal in primary pulmonary hypertension. Exercise speeds up the circulation of blood to the muscles and through the lungs for an adequate oxygen supply. The failure of contracted small pulmonary arteries to dilate during physical exertion in this disease results in a temporary inadequate blood supply to the brain causing a fainting spell.

internist subjected him to a complete examination. This included a complete survey of all his blood chemistry tests and blood count studies, an electrocardiogram, and routine chest X-rays. Nothing was found. Since there was suspicion that the fainting spells were a form of epileptic seizures due to a disease of the central nervous system he was referred to a neurologist. The neurologist made a thorough neurological examination, including an electroencephalogram, which is a standard neurological test that records electric impulses normally produced by the brain. This test shows established normal patterns during sleep and while awake, and it is useful for diagnosing such problems as epilepsy, which are associated with abnormal recordings. All of the studies turned out to be completely normal.

During the patient's vacation in Florida, he decided to renew his old healthy routine and went jogging. He suffered another fainting spell and sought medical care locally. Despite the fact that he never experienced chest pain, the possibility of coronary artery disease was considered, and a coronary angiogram was performed, which was interpreted as showing no significant disease. We have to keep in mind that in those days of the late 1970s the decision to perform a coronary angiogram was not taken lightly, because the test procedure was risky. This procedure was done only prior to some sort of anticipated definitive treatment, such as a coronary bypass operation or coronary angioplasty. In any case, shortly after he returned up north, he died unexpectedly one day while exerting himself physically in some way.

At autopsy we were surprised by his lean and athletic appearance, which seemed incongruous with death. Examination of the heart showed a severe degree of coronary artery arteriosclerosis. One of the two main arteries showed a degree of constriction of the caliber that could have caused the classical complaint of angina pectoris [2], which is chest pain on effort that is relieved by rest. Immediate attention was directed to the angiogram performed earlier, which was recorded on a permanent film. Our staff radiologist reviewed the film and found several easily detectable areas of narrowed arteries due to arteriosclerosis, which matched

---

2. Angina pectoris. This is the classical symptom of severe arteriosclerosis of the two coronary arteries, which supply the heart itself. The disease causes narrowing of the lumens of the arteries with decreased blood flow to heart muscle. This soon lowers the blood flow to an affected region to the degree that the blood supply cannot support the oxygen and sugar essential to the muscular exercise of heartbeats. The early sign is chest pain originating in the deprived region similar to muscular cramps experienced by athletes. The cramps occur when their excessive demands reach a point where the blood supply to their muscles becomes inadequate in spite of a normal blood supply.

the autopsy findings. Obviously, a cardiologist, who may have been inexperienced, had misinterpreted the original angiogram. This led to a failure to take appropriate action, which would have been either a coronary artery bypass or an angioplasty. It must be noted that this case occurred over twenty-five years ago, when the technology of coronary angiography was only ten years old.

The gnawing question was how coronary arteriosclerosis caused fainting spells without the chest pain of angina pectoris. I sought the answer in medical literature and learned that investigators at Montefiore Hospital in New York solved the puzzle about forty years ago. Studies with electrocardiograms during exercise of patients with symptomatic coronary arteriosclerosis revealed that transient very rapid heart rates occurred with ineffective blood flow to the brain and fainting spells without chest pain. Ordinarily, exercise causes rapid heart rates providing higher rates of blood flow throughout the body. However, excessively high heart rates are inefficient, and result in decreased blood flow and consequent fainting. Such rapid rates, called ventricular tachycardia, are dangerous, because they can progress to fatal ventricular fibrillation. This is a state of innumerable asynchronous contractions throughout the heart, which results in a diffuse trembling of the heart wall without effective blood flow and sudden death. For some unknown reason, this patient responded to coronary artery disease with spells of ventricular tachycardia leading to fainting spells without the usual chest pain. This is a rare but currently known manifestation of significant coronary artery disease. Perhaps the decrease in coronary blood flow results in a disturbance of the intrinsic nervous control of the impulses controlling the heart rate, leading to ventricular tachycardia and fatal ventricular fibrillation. The absence of chest pain is unexplained but might be due to the instantaneous loss of consciousness before chest pain can be sensed. Clearly, the correct diagnosis in this case would have led to proper treatment and survival.

22

An Unforgivable Sin

The patient was a woman in her sixties who had smoked for more than forty years. She developed a persistent cough and an X-ray showed a suspicious shadow suggestive of a cancer. The suspicious region was biopsied. A needle aspiration biopsy was done using a long needle on a syringe. The needle was passed through the skin and chest wall into the diseased region of the lung. By applying suction with the syringe, a drop or two of the diseased tissue was aspirated, and then squirted onto a slide. The slide was immediately taken to the laboratory for processing with stains for microscopic study. The aspirated material did contain definite cancer cells. Her physician recommended excision of the cancer with a generous margin of the surrounding lung free of cancer. Before excising the diseased portion of the lung, the surgeon first explored the inner surface of the chest cavity surrounding the lung. He looked for any evidence of spread of the cancer to this surface, which would have meant that surgical cure was impossible and that the operation would be ended. He did find a single suspicious looking nodule, which he cut out and sent for a frozen section.

The frozen section was done by one of my associates, who called me to see it because it was a diagnostic problem. The question was whether this was, indeed, a cancerous nodule or a benign reaction to injury. The tissues lining the inside of the chest cavity can respond to injury such as infection by rapid multiplication of its cells. Such actively proliferating cells often show malignant microscopic changes. I saw no evidence of inflammation. This was a sharply demarcated nodule surrounded by a normal lining and the cells looked like cancer cells. I made a diagnosis of a cancer and the surgeon ended the operation.

The following day when I saw the permanent slides, I was devastated to find that this was not a cancer at all but a wild looking benign change due to some sort of injury. It did have malignant features but the overall pattern was benign. What could the injury be? I then learned that the location of the nodule was where the aspiration biopsy needle pierced the inner surface of the chest cavity before it entered the lung tumor. The injured surface reacted by forming a nodule of proliferating benign cells that mimicked malignant features. The good news was that the lung cancer was still operable for a possible surgical cure.

The error devastated me because infallible medical practice was my standard and I felt disgraced. I was overwhelmed by remorse and guilt for causing the pain that the patient and family suffered by being told that the cancer was inoperable and for subjecting the patient to a second operation. To add salt to the injury, this patient was also the wife of a physician on our staff. They were warm friends, whose social company we enjoyed regularly. I nearly died as I contemplated what I had done, and immediately sought her husband to tell him what happened. I explained what happened and his first reaction was that she was operable after all. He made no critical appraisal of my error and made no reconciling comments. He was older than me, which helped because older physicians appreciate best that the only way to avoid errors is not to practice medicine.

The surgeon was obviously upset. He knew that this was not the first or last time that he would have to deal with an inaccurate frozen section diagnosis. He did not go so far as to condemn me for avoidable negligence.

Several days later, the patient's internist visited me to tell me that the error was probably a blessing. He noted that she had difficulties breathing after the original operation due to retained mucous secretions in her lungs. Lifelong smokers commonly develop chronic emphysema and bronchitis, which cause excessive mucous secretions into the airways with difficulty in breathing. This interval was a welcome opportunity to clear her lungs and improve function to better prepare her for the second operation, which would remove part of one lung. She underwent the second operation successfully. Unfortunately, she died several months later of spread of the cancer to other organs.

Several years later, in 1989, I heard a talk by a well-known pathologist at a conference on diagnostic errors revealed by postmortem examinations. The panelist was Dr. Rolla B. Hill, a leading American pathologist and an advocate of the autopsy, which had steadily declined in number since the 1970s. He presented the idea that unavoidable errors without negligence were inevitable, and indeed necessary, because the only way to avoid errors was by ending medical practice altogether. He cited the work of two fellows of the Hastings Center, a think tank in Westchester County, New York. They were Drs. Samuel Gorovitz and Alasdair McIntyre, who proposed a theory of medical fallibility, which they attributed to two factors. One was the vast void in medical knowledge. The other factor is unfamiliar and can be expressed in various ways. In a nutshell, the other factor is Nature, which delights in surprising us by ignoring our books with endless unpredictable ways of doing as she pleases. When I heard these ideas, I sensed sunshine breaking through clouds, and a heavy burden of guilt lifted off my back. My remorse was unaffected because of the permanent question, "What if?" The answer to this question is unknowable but asking it suggests possible fault. It would be ideal if Nature were obliging and presided over bad outcomes that were clearly due to either negligent malpractice or unavoidable factors. There are endless shades of gray between these black and white extremes.

23

A Delayed Bomb

Early in 1980, a Haitian woman in her forties was admitted to the hospital with increasing difficulty in breathing of several days duration. She also complained about itchy patches of skin rashes on her arms and body, which spread over the past few weeks. She was admitted directly to the intensive care unit because she had fever and was gasping for air on admission. She was immediately given oxygen and put on a respirator with some relief. A chest X-ray revealed extensive shadows in both lungs due to pneumonia of some sort. Examination of her sputum for the usual bacteria causing pneumonia was negative. A dermatologist examined the rash and suggested a biopsy. The biopsy revealed a rare type of cancer of the immune system called a lymphoma. The difficulty in breathing worsened over the next few days in spite of the oxygen and respirator treatment. This meant that whatever was afflicting the lungs was progressively filling all the air spaces in the same way that water fills the air spaces in death due to drowning. There was no response to intravenous antibiotic treatment. She slipped into coma after several days and died shortly thereafter.

At autopsy, the skin rashes looked deceptively benign because the skin was not thickened. Pneumonia involved both lungs, which made them feel solid like a mattress rather than the normal consistency of a soft feather pillow. They were dark red in contrast to the normal light pink. Each lung weighed about two pounds, three times heavier than normal. This is the maximum weight possible with any lung disease, which replaces the air in the air spaces. Bacteria and pus in bacterial pneumonia, or cancer cells arising in the lungs or spreading there from other organs, may also fill these air spaces. This was an obvious pneumonia but the failure to find any of the usual bacteria in the sputum made us impatient to see how the disease appeared under the microscope. I eagerly studied the slides the following day and I was surprised to see the features of a curious and very rare cause of pneumonia, which I had seen only once before during my training days. Dr. H.M. Zimmerman had a collection of interesting slides of rare diseases, which he showed to his residents and it included the disease in this case. It has no common name familiar to the laity and is named after the organism that causes it, Pneumocystis carinii pneumonia (PCP).

What makes the microscopic appearance so distinctive is the material that fills the air spaces. It appears foamy because of the tiny bubbles it contains. Nothing else looks quite the same. Special stains reveal that the tiny bubbles are actually the infectious organisms, a kind of fungus that grows in the air spaces. I had no idea why she developed this rare infection. We all wondered whether the associated lymphoma of the skin, another rare disease, might have had something to do with it.

This patient proved to be my first contact with Adult Immune Deficiency Syndrome (AIDS) due to the virus called the Human Immunodeficiency Disease Virus (HIV). This is the scourge of the late twentieth century and our times. AIDS was unknown when I did this autopsy and was described as a new infectious disease several months later due to a virus that kills cells of the immune system[1]. Victims are prone to infections of all the usual sorts and also infections by usually harmless organisms. There are many harmless bacteria and fungi that are normal inhabitants of our alimentary system from the mouth to the anus. We live at peace with them and actually depend on some for their production of beneficial chemicals. Wiping out all the bacteria in the intestines with antibiotics can lead to a bleeding tendency because some produce vitamin K, which is required for blood to clot normally. Apparently, our intact immune systems are what keep these organisms harmless. The causative organism of PCP is a normal inhabitant of our mouths and grows wild when HIV destroys the immune system. PCP was a common cause of death in patients with AIDS. A drug called bactrim prevents this infection in AIDS patients today. Bactrim and other new drugs have contributed to the prolonged life spans of these patients. There are still many other bacteria and fungi, which can grow wild, and for which there is no effective treatment. Advances in drugs that inhibit the growth of HIV with restoration of the immune system have been very effective, but not yet curative. The rare type of lymphoma in this case is also characteristic of AIDS, which is a predisposing factor.

I was shaken somewhat when I realized months later that I had been exposed to infection, but took comfort in being free of symptoms. The risk of pathologists acquiring infections during autopsies has always existed. They may acquire tuberculosis and I know of deaths of three physicians, including one young intern and

---

1. See Appendix B.

two pathologists. They died of viral diseases of the liver acquired from infected patients. AIDS constantly posed a danger of being undiagnosed in a patient dying of something else, such as a viral infection of the liver due to drug addiction acquired by using contaminated needles. Contaminated needles can transmit both viral infections of the liver and AIDS. These risks led to the adoption of techniques called universal precautions to protect pathologists and their assistants. The techniques were recommended for all autopsies and were basically operating room precautions, which protect the patient and the surgeon. The new precautions did protect the pathologist and assistants but are not the equivalent of operating room standards. The walls and floors of operating rooms are completely disinfected after surgery. This is impossible in most autopsy rooms, which are usually cluttered with equipment and stored supplies making floor and wall space inaccessible to disinfecting methods.

It is no exaggeration that some pathologists were terrified by the prospect of doing an autopsy on known AIDS cases and refused to do them. I never condoned such refusals because becoming a pathologist entails more risk of acquired infections than other specialties, and it is unethical to evade this responsibility in risky cases. As a practical matter, universal precautions do protect the pathologist adequately enough to eliminate immobilizing fear.

The coming of AIDS as a global catastrophe is a unique event in our lifetime. Hindsight of other great epidemics, which have come and gone over the centuries, illustrate the grand design of nature in directing the genesis of new forms of life, including some that can cause deadly diseases.

1990–2000, The University of Connecticut Health Center, Farmington, Connecticut, Associate Professor of Pathology

24

A Devastating Pregnancy

In spite of all the revolutionary advances in medical knowledge, the flow of baffling cases persisted and actually seemed more frequent at the University of Connecticut Health Center during the 1990s. This was undoubtedly due to its status as a tertiary hospital, which attracted patients with unusual problems. It was better staffed and equipped to manage difficult cases than average community hospitals. After more than forty years of experience, I was constantly as surprised by diseases I never saw before as I was as a trainee. The eagerness of my students matched mine in studying strange diseases and made me feel like I was one of them. The following example of a mysterious and fatal heart disease was typical.

The patient was a Hispanic woman, twenty-three years of age who was admitted because of increasing shortness of breath and swelling of the legs of about one week's duration. She had delivered her third baby about ten days before. Although her first two pregnancies were normal, the recent one was marked by episodes of transient difficulties in breathing, typical of asthmatic attacks, which began in the sixth month of pregnancy. Persistent and increasing difficulty in breathing continued several days after delivery, and was followed by gradual swelling of the legs, beginning around the ankles.

The physical examination showed signs typical of full blown heart failure. The blood pressure was low, 80/50, the pulse was rapid, 110, and she was breathing rapidly. The sounds of excess water in the lungs were heard with the stethoscope. The temperature was slightly elevated to 99 degrees and the legs were swollen because of excessive water accumulation. She received ACE-inhibitors and Beta-blockers[1], which usually relieve progressive heart failure. She did not respond to any of these treatments and got progressively worse.

Imaging studies of the heart showed normal heart valves and weak contractions of all parts of the heart. This indicated an impairment of all of the heart muscle by some disease, which was of unknown cause.

In the medical community, when doctors have no idea of the cause of heart failure in an occasional case, they apply a diagnosis of "cardiomyopathy," which simply means that there is an unknown disease of the heart muscle. This may sound pointless, but it has the sole value of agreeing on one term for general medical use that defines a working diagnosis recognized by all. For example, this was the diagnosis actually used when the request for a heart transplant was made, which was her only hope for cure.

A biopsy of the heart muscle was taken to determine whether there was a cause for heart failure that could be treated. The microscopic study showed normal looking muscle. An electron microscopic study was also done, which increases the magnification of what is seen under the ordinary microscope a thousand times. This often exposes obvious disease not seen under ordinary microscopic study, but was completely normal looking in this case. I never saw an electron microscopic study before that was of no help in a difficult disease.

The patient was transferred to the intensive care unit about a week before she died, without responding to life support on respirators, and drugs. The autopsy findings in the heart were baffling, because it was only slightly dilated but otherwise normal, as far as its muscular walls, the valves, and the coronary arteries were concerned. Microscopic studies of many samples were again disappointing.

In contrast to the lack of diagnostic changes in the heart, the changes in the lungs, liver, and intestines due to heart failure were as severe as they can possibly get [2]. These days, these severe changes are seen less often because of the effectiveness of the drugs used to treat heart failure. Of course, patients with successfully treated heart failure may later die of other complications.

This case was another instance of a complete void in medical knowledge. It is a very rare but recognized complication of pregnancy known as a "peripartum cardiomyopathy." The heart uniquely shows normal structures in the face of unresponsive heart failure. I never knew there was such a disease until I studied

---

1. These two drugs were successfully developed to eliminate hypertension and are still in use. Doctors treating hypertension in patients with heart failure realized that the drugs had an unexpected beneficial effect on heart failure. Exactly how these drugs have such a near miraculous effect is not known and is under investigation. (See Appendix A).

this case. I was amazed by the severity of the changes because of the short duration of the severe heart failure. I wondered whether the development of asthma in her sixth month of pregnancy was actually due to the onset of heart failure, which can behave in this fashion.

It is interesting that heart specialists at the National Institutes of Health published a report on this rare disease in recent years. Their purpose was to explain the need for all cases to be gathered in a registry to get a more complete picture of all its features for a better understanding. Some cases do survive, and it would benefit all future cases to learn how the survivors differed from the fatal cases.

---

2. These severe changes were seen often in young patients dying of heart failure due to rheumatic heart disease many years ago ending in the 1960s (See Appendix A). Heart failure was caused by permanent deformities of the heart valves that followed repeated attacks of joint pains in acute rheumatic fever. As one pathologist described in his book comparing the long-term effects of these attacks on the joints and the heart, "Acute rheumatic fever licks the joints and bites the heart." The permanent deformities of the heart valves were due to progressive obstruction by scarring. For example, the mitral valve is made up of two delicate leaflets of thin tissues which together open and close the opening of the valve. The opening normally measures more than an inch in diameter when the leaflets part to permit newly oxygenated blood from the lungs to enter the heart for distribution to the body. All of the circulating blood must pass through this valve with every heartbeat. Rheumatic heart disease resulted in thickened and fused rigid valves, which constricted the mitral valve opening to less than ¼ inch in diameter. The pathologic change is called mitral stenosis and has been aptly described as a buttonhole valve. The unmistakable changes in the lungs, liver, and intestines are due to engorgement of these organs by blood backed up by the constricted valve over many years.

25

Sudden Death

This 40-year-old woman suffered from an uncommon disease that is well known by physicians. It has no common name familiar to the public. It was formerly called "scleroderma" (Greek, *scleros* meaning hard, and *derma* meaning skin) because it caused thickening and hardening of the skin. These changes occur slowly over months. The joints become steadily stiffened and painful as the skin hardens. The diagnosis is not obvious at first until the telltale skin changes occur. In recent years, another name was introduced for this disease, namely "systemic sclerosis," because it was not confined to the skin, but also internal organs including the heart, lungs, kidneys, and intestines.

This is one of many baffling diseases of unknown cause. It is due to the excessive action of an otherwise normal cell in the makeup of our tissues. The cell is called a fibroblast, which is a key player in our bodies because it makes a tough microscopic fiber called collagen, which holds our organs together. It is also the major component of scar tissue following a healed injury. If we eliminate all the cells in the body, and just preserve the bundles of collagen fibers, you would still see the outlines of every bodily structure clearly, because of the remaining collagen framework. An analogy would be the framework of a house. The fibroblasts are normally dormant in fully-grown adults and somehow become activated in this disease to produce excessive collagen. The result is stiffening and thickening of tissues, and the relentless entrapment of the cells of an organ by engulfing layers of excessive collagen. The entrapped cells are, in a sense, buried alive and slowly die, as they are isolated from the nearest blood supply for oxygen and nutrients.

The deadly entrapment of small organs in skin such as hair follicles and sweat glands results in the loss of hair and dry skin. The diffuse overgrowth of collagen fibers between the muscle cells in the heart may eventually cause heart failure. The thickening of the walls of the air sacs in the lungs may increase to the point of fatal impairment of the ability of the blood to absorb oxygen. The disease attacks the muscular walls of the intestines impairing their undulating contractions that carry its contents forward. These patients often develop difficulty in swallowing due to the destruction of the muscles in the esophagus, the tube that passes down the chest from the mouth to the stomach. Involvement of the kidneys results in severe hypertension and kidney failure.

This patient first developed stiffened and painful joints about two and a half years before her death. Difficulty in swallowing followed by tightening of the skin ensued during the next half year. She was then referred to a rheumatologist, who made the diagnosis of systemic sclerosis. She received a variety of drugs, which might help, such as steroids and D-penicillamine, but all failed to halt the progression of disease.

She was first seen at UCHC three months before her death as a candidate for a blood stem cell transplant. This was purely an experimental treatment based on the theory that the cause of the disease was an abnormality of the immune system. The cells of the immune system make all sorts of proteins that help us kill harmful foreign invaders such as bacteria, and to neutralize harmful substances. One of the many proteins they make is one that stimulates fibroblasts to become active and make collagen. This is a beneficial effect in the healing of any injury. The theory is that somehow this effect is rampant in systemic sclerosis because of an uncontrolled production of this substance by outlaw cells of the immune system. One possible way of stopping the disease is to wipe out all the cells of the immune system including the outlaws. There are normally stem cells of the immune system in the blood, which are the potential seeds for the growth of a brand new immune system. These special cells are harvested from the patient's blood and then preserved in a frozen state. A combination of powerful drugs is then given to the patient to wipe out the existing immune system including the outlaw cells. Antibiotics are given to protect the patient from infections, which are deadly without a working immune system. A transfusion of the patient's own preserved stem cells is then given with the intent for them to "be fruitful, and multiply" in order to establish a new healthy immune system.

Powerful drugs are used to do this, followed by a transfusion of the patient's own preserved stem cells, which would be the seeds of a restored hopefully normal immune system. She underwent this procedure and had the transfusion of her stem cells two weeks before her death. Her peripheral blood count showed an expected complete absence of cells of the immune system for a week. The new cells then appeared and the counts of immune cells reached normal levels in a few days. She was treated with powerful antibiotics during this critical time of being susceptible to all sorts of infections. Her progress was very encouraging. The stem cell transplant was an obvious success. She was seen as an outpatient in the transplant clinic for a scheduled routine visit on the day of her death. Everything was going well and she left with an appointment for a future routine visit. As her husband was driving out of the parking lot, she suddenly lost consciousness and slumped in her seat. He quickly drove back to the nearby emergency room, where she was pronounced dead on arrival. The shocked husband readily gave consent for an autopsy.

The heart presented striking changes at autopsy. It was normal in size but was extremely flabby in contrast to its usual firm consistency. It was unusual for this organ, which usually maintains its shape after death to appear flattened out like a collapsed balloon. The other surprising change was its color, which I had never seen before. The heart wall is normally dark red in contrast to this patient's heart, which was brown and streaked throughout by light tan stripes. The appearance was like the stripes of a tiger. Indeed, this change was described in our books as "tigering of the heart," which typically occurred in a disease called pernicious anemia[1]. This was not a case of pernicious anemia, which I had also never seen because it was largely eliminated as a cause of death about sixty years ago when successful treatment with liver extract was discovered. The disease was due to vitamin B-12 deficiency, which was the curative ingredient in liver extract.

A special chemical test was done on the heart to determine whether death of the heart muscle had occurred during life, such as happens with a typical heart attack. We were amazed to find scattered areas of dead muscle roughly corresponding to the light tan streaks. This finding baffled us because there was no hint of heart failure before she died. The only symptom of heart problems was an abnormal heart rhythm she showed eight days before death. An appropriate drug successfully returned the heart to a normal rhythm. It was as if the heart were overwhelmed during a short time before death by a powerful poison. Her last hemoglobin count two days before death was 8 units as compared to a normal of 15 units. This indicated an anemia associated with a recovering bone marrow following powerful chemotherapy but was perfectly compatible with life. Systemic sclerosis was clearly not a cause of the changes in her heart. The cause of these

---

1. Pernicious anemia over a period of several years resulted in a slow progressive decrease in the number of circulating red blood cells. They contain hemoglobin, the vital protein that carries oxygen from the lungs to the tissue, and the concentration of blood hemoglobin gradually fell over a few years from normal levels of 15 units to 1.5 units terminally, which caused death. The cause of the disease eventually was discovered to be a deficiency of vitamin B-12. The "tigering of the heart" was attributed to long-standing severe anemia.

deadly changes in the heart remains unknown. Neither the heart nor kidneys showed evidence of the overproduction of collagen associated with systemic sclerosis. The remainder of the autopsy did show evidence of the disease in the skin, lungs, esophagus, and intestines.

26

The Doctors Never Heard of This One

A 54-year-old man was admitted to the emergency room complaining of severe pain of his muscles and bones unrelieved by drugs. He was alert but pale and sweating profusely. His medical history indicated that he had developed a lymphoma three years before, a cancer of the immune system. He responded to treatment with powerful drugs and was free of disease until a month ago when enlarged lymph nodes recurred in an armpit due to the lymphoma. He received a full course of treatment ending ten days prior to his admission to the emergency room. He was treated with morphine for the intractable pain and admitted to the hospital.

He complained that his pains felt like the bends[1], which he had experienced as a scuba diver when rising to the water surface too quickly. Blood tests indicated that he was suffering from a systemic formation of small blood clots, which could produce bends and even death if there was a critical loss of blood flow to vital organs. There is a well-known deadly disease that is the result of widespread clotting of blood in small blood vessels. Its cause is unknown but an effective treatment is to replace all the plasma, which is the liquid component of blood, with transfused plasma from blood donations. This radical treatment is based on the

---

1. The bends are due to the passage of nitrogen dissolved in blood into a gaseous phase forming bubbles. Nitrogen is normally dissolved in the blood and is carried along with oxygen since 4/5ths of the air we breathe is nitrogen. The problem is that blood absorbs more nitrogen when the body is subjected to the high pressures of deep water in addition to the normal atmospheric air pressure. Bends occur when the change to normal atmospheric pressure is too rapid and the excess nitrogen bubbles out of solution in the blood. The bubbles are dangerous because they obstruct blood flow in small vessels, which supply all tissues including muscles. Muscles become very painful when deprived of a blood supply and the deprivation of blood flow to vital organs can be deadly.

presumption that an abnormal component of the patient's plasma is the culprit. This treatment was administered twice to the patient with no effect. The patient grew steadily worse, went into coma, and died about one week after the onset of muscle pains.

At autopsy, careful examination of the lymph nodes and all the organs revealed no persistent cancerous cells. These structures showed the effects of the powerful drugs he had received to destroy the recurrent cancer ending about two weeks before death. The affected lymph nodes did show devastation as if a storm had blown away most of the cells.

Microscopic studies of the other organs showed an amazing change. Most of the small microscopic blood vessels called capillaries, which deliver blood to each cell, were stuffed with clear bubbles, which also appeared in some of the larger blood vessels. One of the possible reasons for these bubbles was that they were droplets of fat, the same as oil droplets of any kind. Fat is suspected when we see round clear bubbly spaces and this can easily be tested with a special dye called "oil red O" which is soluble in oil. The chemically untreated tissue block is frozen and a thin slice of it is cut, put on a slide, and bathed in the "oil red O." The only thing on the slide that will take the stain and appear bright red is a fat or oil droplet.

As we expected, all of the bubbles in blood vessels were, indeed, stained bright red proving that they were fat droplets. This was easily seen in the lungs, kidneys, heart, brain, and muscles. The blockage of countless microscopic capillaries explained the muscle pains identical to bends and the fatal outcome because vital organs, particularly the heart, lungs, and brain were affected. Such oil droplets circulating in the blood are called "fat emboli" and the disease is called "fat embolization."

Where could so much fat come from? All pathologists see a few fat emboli at autopsy occasionally in patients who die for any reason, and who also had a recent fractured bone such as a fractured hip in the elderly. Presumably, the droplets of fat are released into the bloodstream from disrupted fat cells, which normally pack the bone marrow spaces. This sort of fat emboli differs from those seen in this patient because they also contain bits of disrupted bone marrow tissue. This case was different because there were no fractures or bits of marrow and the fat embolization was massive. It overwhelmed capillaries everywhere and shut off the blood supply eventually to vital organs. Where did all this fat come from? The frustrating answer is that we don't know for sure. This case was an example of an extremely rare event called "atraumatic fat embolization" because fat emboli occur in the absence of fractured bones. The rare cases are characterized by some kind of antecedent stress, such as shock for any reason. The side effects of the drug treatment for cancer were the possible factors in this case.

An inkling of how this could happen is suggested by a case of fatal massive fat embolization due to multiple fractures, which I saw during my early training years at Montefiore Hospital. A patient in his fifties killed himself by jumping out of a window of the third floor of the pavilion for private patients. He fell on a concrete pavement and lived for a short time before he was finally pronounced dead. He had an operation several days before his death, which revealed an inoperable cancer of the pancreas. The tumor had already spread to the liver, which was peppered by numerous small cancerous nodules. He was driven to suicide after he learned that his death was certain.

The autopsy confirmed the cancer of the pancreas, which had spread to lymph nodes, the liver, and lungs. There were also numerous fractured bones from the fall. The microscopic findings were striking because there was massive fat embolization as in the patient discussed above with one difference. In addition to pure fat emboli, the lungs also showed numerous microscopic bits of bone marrow in small blood vessels. These were carried to the lungs in the bloodstream when the fractures fragmented the marrow and pushed bits into ruptured blood vessels. The marrow emboli were fragments of intact normal fatty marrow with normal islands of blood forming cells.

While it was obvious that the bone marrow emboli in the suicidal patient were due to fractures, the big question then was also: Where did all the free fat droplets come from? It seemed then that the obvious answer was that the disrupted fatty tissue in the fractures released both the fat droplets and the fragments of marrow. Dr. Zimmerman dismissed this idea because the problem was that the distribution of free fat emboli everywhere in the circulating blood was simply too much to explain by ruptured fat cells from a fragmented marrow. Dr. Zimmerman then explained to us that the fragments of marrow bits in the lungs are commonly seen in anyone who has had a recent fractured bone, as I noted before. These cases do not show the extent of free circulating fat seen in this case. He went on to explain that this fatal phenomenon can actually occur in the absence of any fractures and that the explanation was unknown.

He cited a reference, which was published about twenty-five years before in the 1920s, which drew attention to the possibility of massive fat embolization without multiple fractures. I read the reference, which discussed the relationship of stress to the development of fat emboli. Dr. Zimmerman pointed out that multiple fractures are one form of severe stress and that most of the pure fat emboli might very well be another example of stress causing "atraumatic" fat embolization in a patient where the stress causing shock happened to be multiple fractures.

How this happens is still unknown but an understanding of how fat is normally handled in the body does suggest a possible way. The total amount of fat normally present in blood varies with meals but averages about 10 grams or 1/3 ounce. The normal total body fat content is about 15% in men, and 22% in women, who are not overweight. A man weighing 170 pounds would then have about 25 pounds of total body fat, which is about twelve hundred times the amount in the blood at any one time. The blood fat is not static but being actively transported from one place to another. The cycle begins in the intestine, where about 100 grams or 3 1/3 ounces of fat are digested with food daily. All of this fat is transported to the liver, and the fat depots for storage, which are most prominent under the skin. The liver and the fat depots, in turn, return fat to the blood for delivery to all the organs, which utilize fat in many ways. Fat is leaving and entering the blood constantly without forming fat emboli because of the way it is carried in the blood. Fat is insoluble in blood water.

Nature overcomes this difficulty in an amazing way by packaging the fat as tiny quantities completely enclosed in a water-friendly shell. The shell is impervious to the fat and is made of a combination of a protein and a special fat called a lipoprotein. The intestinal cells absorb digested fat and package it in tiny quantities within the lipoprotein shells. The packages of fat are called chylomicrons and are secreted into the blood. The fat is delivered to the liver for processing and to the fat storage depots for storage of excess fat. Fat is normally transported as chylomicrons to all the organs both as a fuel for energy and as a necessary component of special cell structures.

The chylomicrons first adhere to the surfaces of the target cells. The transfer of the fat from within the chylomicron to the inside of a cell is done by a complex stepwise process, which prevents contact of the fat with blood at any time. There is a dynamic constant circulation of chylomicrons between the intestines, the liver, fat depots, and all organs dependent on the integrity of the chylomicron. It is conceivable that an interference with how cells make a chylomicron shell, or something that ruptures it, could result in the continuous pouring of free fat into the circulation. This is like injecting oil into a vein, which would also produce deadly droplets occluding capillaries. It is conceivable our patient's muscle pains and consequent death was due to fat embolization caused by ruptured chylomicrons. This is an interesting theory but then a big question still remains. Exactly what makes chylomicron shells rupture in rare cases of severe stress? The answer is probably worth a Nobel Prize.

Conclusion

During my career as a pathologist, I was involved in about 7,500 autopsies and saw about 150,000 surgical specimens and biopsies. The twenty-six anecdotes presented here concerned unusual patients. Each one taught me more than any other 100 autopsies or 1,000 surgical specimens ever could. If other pathologists recorded memoirs of their respective experiences, I would guess that each of them would have had a similar number of unusual cases, but perhaps far different from my own. In fact, if ten or more pathologists got together at the end of their careers to combine their recorded experiences with problem cases into one book, it is likely that most of the cases would prove to be unique, like the shapes of clouds or fingerprints. This is one basis for recognizing the inherent uncertainties of medical practice, including pathology.

Since all of the experiences presented here were diagnostic problems, including some with poor outcomes, the reader might acquire a sense of insecurity about whether it is ever possible to get quality medical care. To respond to that concern, I have to point out that these cases represent a very small fraction of all cases seen by doctors. There really is no way to measure the degree of uncertainty in medical practice, which may result in mismanagement. However, the fraction is probably very small and of a magnitude less than 1%. For example, the twenty-six anecdotes cited here were recalled in hindsight from a total experience with about 82,500 cases, and thus comprise only 0.03%. The remaining cases are not discussed here because they presented no problems. The current frequency of unavoidable errors revealed by autopsy reviews is summarized in the Appendix[1]. Two examples of the more common errors are also discussed[2]. The Appendix also contains the findings of studies, which indicate that traditional bedside methods are actually more diagnostically helpful than the new technologies[3].

In conclusion, I emphasize three major problems that have to be solved in order to end the current storm of medical litigation and its devastating effects on medical care standards and education. One is to end the delusion of medical

---

1. See Appendix C.
2. See Appendix D.
3. See Appendix E.

infallibility shared by the public and many doctors. Another is to have alternative sources of compensation for patient injury due to medical error other than or in addition to doctors' liability insurance, the current sole source of compensation for all errors, avoidable and unavoidable. The third issue is our flawed legal system for dealing with patient injury. Relying on lay juries swayed by persuasive trial lawyers has led to astronomical injury awards and skyrocketing medical liability insurance premiums. We need to replace the current legal system with a panel system composed of physicians, lawyers, the clergy, and informed lay members. Such panels would evaluate litigated cases and recommend both fair and rational compensation for plaintiffs, as well as sanctions for culpable doctors.

I have emphasized Nature's role in contributing to our fallibility. I would like to close with a reverent tribute to Nature for her role in more than balancing the uncertainties of medical practice with her incredible and endless healing powers.

PART III

Appendix

A. The Heart, Circulatory System, and Heart Failure

The heart is a lifelong pump, which maintains the circulation of blood to all organs. Glucose and oxygen are essential for life. Glucose, a component of ordinary sugar, is the basic fuel of the body. A fuel is needed for a constant source of heat that maintains the normal body temperature at 98.6 degrees Fahrenheit. This temperature is a measure of the amount of heat energy required to drive the countless chemical reactions that keep us alive. Oxygen has the same role in the body as it does in feeding a fire of burning wood. It "burns" glucose similarly in a chemical way but without flames.

Glucose contains units of two elements, carbon and hydrogen. These two units are broken off the glucose molecule in a series of chemical reactions, which result in every carbon and hydrogen unit being combined with oxygen to produce two well-known products, carbon dioxide and water. An infinitesimally small amount of heat is generated with each separation of a carbon or hydrogen unit from the glucose molecule. This steady heat production in tiny ovens in some 70 trillion cells maintains our normal body temperature. This is how the "burning" of glucose produces carbon dioxide and water the same way as burning wood, but without flames.

Both land dwelling animals and fish require oxygen for life support. The air we breathe contains an abundant source of oxygen, which our circulating blood extracts in the lungs. Fish "breathe" by constantly sucking water through their mouths and out over their gills, which extract the free oxygen dissolved in water into their circulating blood.

Nature has designed the anatomy of the circulatory system to maintain a continuous supply of oxygen to all organs from the surrounding air for land animals and from the water for fish. Studying the fish heart and circulatory system will be helpful to understand the anatomy of the human heart. Blood vessels with thin walls called veins deliver blood from all organs to the relaxed heart, which then contracts and expels blood to all organs through blood vessels with thicker walls called arteries. Arteries have thicker walls than veins because the circulating blood in them is under a higher pressure, which is generated by the pumping action of heartbeats propelling blood flow to all organs. The fish heart has two main chambers (See Figure 4).

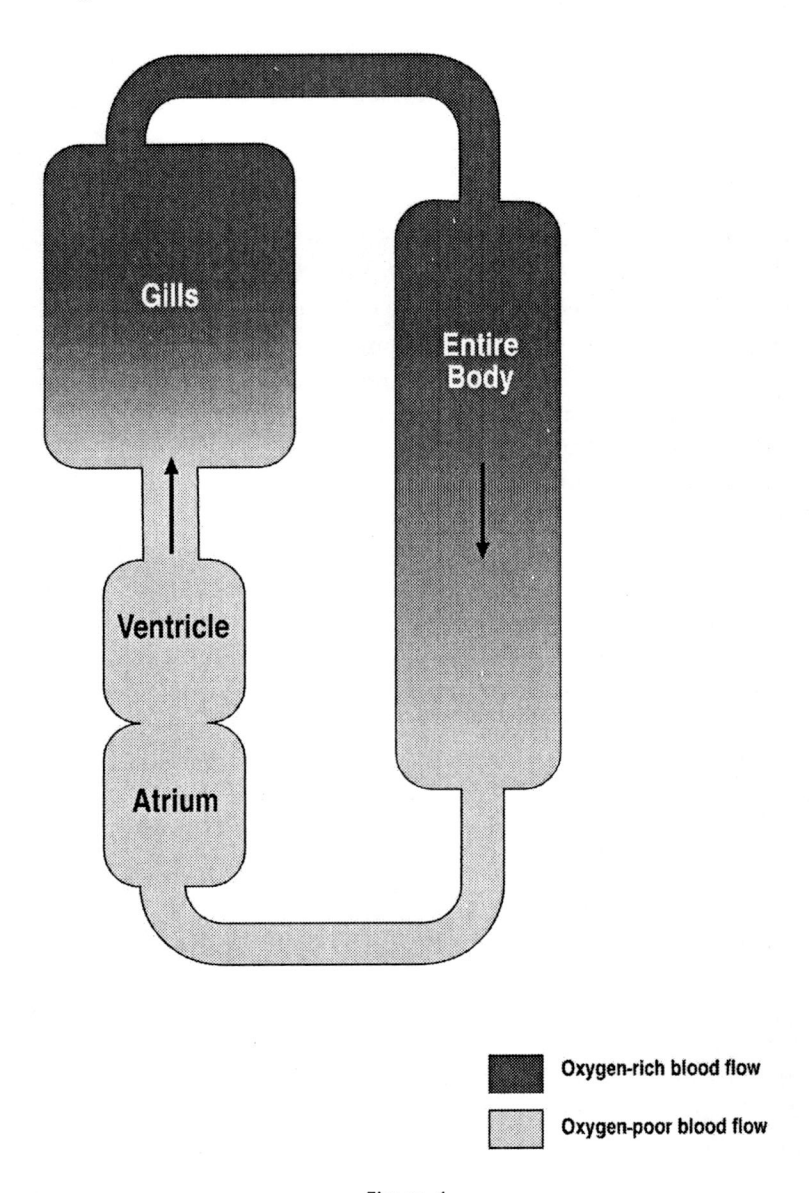

Figure 4

One, the atrium receives venous blood low in oxygen from the body. The blood passes into the second connecting chamber, the ventricle, which propels the blood out of the heart into arteries, which enter the gills. The arteries branch repeatedly into progressively smaller branches into millions of microscopic blood vessels called capillaries, which have walls one cell thick. The oxygen carried in blood is transported in special cells called red blood cells, which give blood its familiar red color. These cells are very small. A chain of 900 red blood cells would be only ¼ inch long. The diameters of capillaries are about the same as red blood cells, which must pass through them in single file. Each red blood cell picks up its oxygen load from oxygen dissolved in the water passing through the fish's mouth and out through its gill slits. Each unit of oxygen passes through the single cell layer forming the capillary wall and into the red cell within. The capillaries with a fresh supply of oxygenated blood repeatedly join together to form progressively larger arteries, which eventually join to form a single large artery, which branches repeatedly to supply all the organs. These oxygen-rich vessels form millions of capillaries in organs where red blood cells unload their oxygen through the capillary walls to supply cells of surrounding organs. The capillaries then form veins carrying oxygen-poor blood back to the heart for recycling.

The human heart is, in a sense, a combination of two fish hearts, one on the right side and the other on the left (See Figure 5).

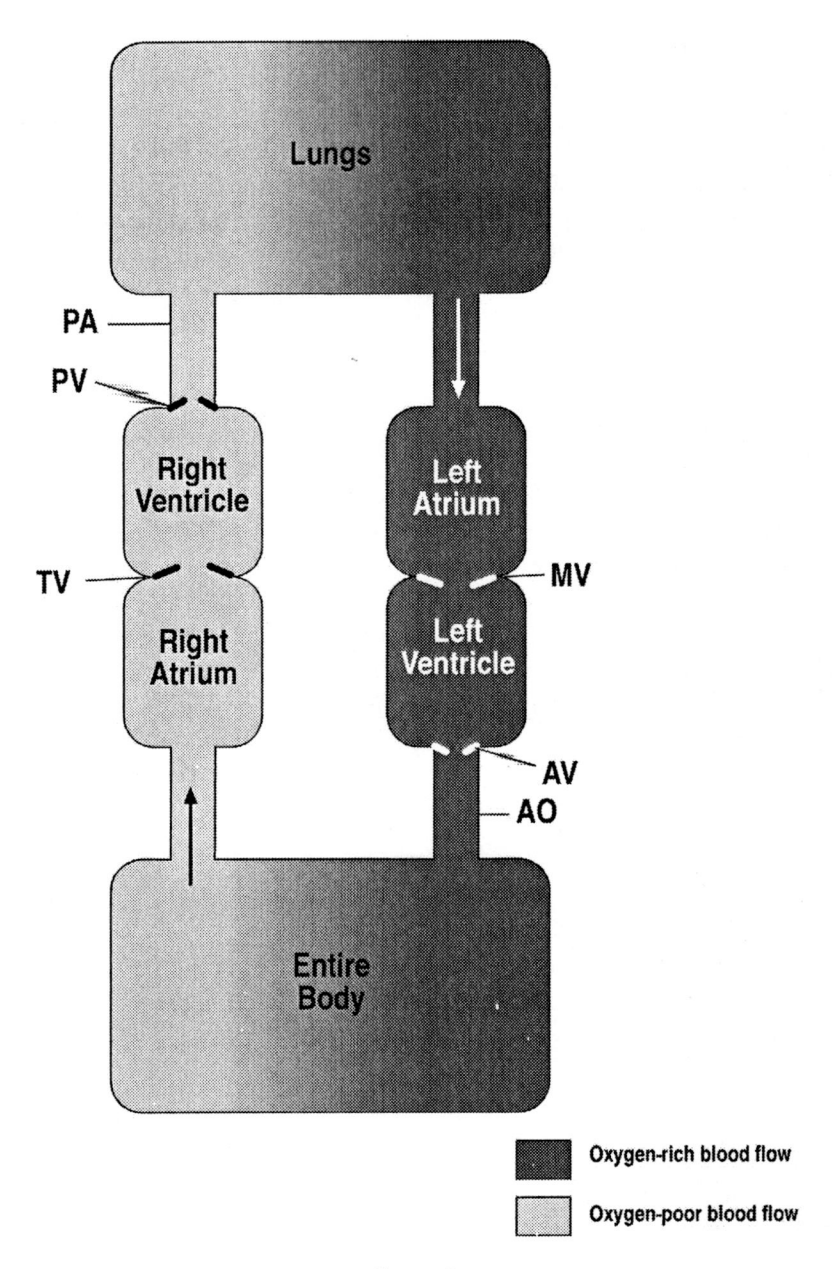

Figure 5

There is a right atrium (Fig. 5 RA) and ventricle (Fig. 5 RV) and a left atrium (Fig. 5 LA) and ventricle (Fig. 5 LV); a heart with four chambers. The right atrium receives venous blood from the entire body and passes it through the tricuspid valve (Fig. 5 TV)[1] into the right ventricle. The ventricle contracts with each heartbeat and propels blood through the pulmonary valve (Fig. 5 PV) into a short, large artery, called the pulmonary aorta (Fig. 5 PA), which divides into a branch to each lung, where it forms a network of millions of capillaries lining millions of air sacs. Oxygen units in inspired air pass through a single cell layer lining the air sacs to enter red blood cells passing through capillaries in single file. The oxygen-rich capillaries join to form veins, which join one another to form two large pulmonary veins from each lung, which drain directly into the left atrium (Fig. 5 LA). The blood then passes through the mitral valve (Fig. 5 MV) into the left ventricle, which contracts and pumps blood through the aortic valve (Fig. 5 AV) into the aorta (Fig. 5 AO). This is a large main artery as big as a garden hose, which gives off branches to the entire body forming a network of millions of capillaries releasing oxygen from red cells into tissues. The capillaries then form veins, which eventually join to form two large veins, which drain into the right atrium.

The filling of the two atriums, the passage of the blood into the two ventricles, and the expulsion of blood into the lungs from the right ventricle, and to the entire body from the left ventricle all happen simultaneously. Normally, the two ventricles each pump out an equal volume of blood with each heartbeat.

Heart Failure

Normally, each ventricle ejects between one half and three-quarters of the contained blood load with each heartbeat, and the ejected amounts from each one are normally equal. The residues remaining in the ventricles after each contraction are normal. Heart failure occurs when the amount of residual blood in either or both ventricles exceeds more than half of the load just before contraction. This only occurs when there is some sort of injury to the heart preventing sufficiently forceful contractions. The injury may be a discrete loss of contracting heart muscle affecting either or both ventricles as occurs in a heart attack. The injury may affect the entire heart causing weaker contractions as occurs in virus infections of the heart. Another injurious change may be a bottleneck narrowing of a valve opening due to disease. Attacks of acute rheumatic fever in children and young

---

1. All the valves act as one-way valves, opening only to permit blood flow in one direction.

adults are serious because of permanent injury to the valves of the heart. This disease is of unknown cause. Each attack causes partial destruction with inflammation and scarring of one or more valves. For example, the opening of the mitral valve between the left atrium and ventricle is large enough to admit a golf ball. Imagine scarring reducing the opening to a slit the size of a buttonhole. Imagine a similar deformity of the valve opening between the left ventricle and aorta, which is normally perfectly round with a diameter of about an inch. The left ventricle will get larger to generate a more forceful contraction. There is a limit to how large the ventricle can get to overcome the increasing narrowing of the opening. Eventually, it fails to expel a normal volume of blood with each contraction with an increasing residual load, in addition to the continuing constant load from the left atrium. This inability of a ventricle to pump out a normal volume of blood introduces abnormalities, which are characteristic of heart failure.

The blood supply to all organs including all muscles is depressed causing weakness and a feeling of being too tired to continue a normal activity like walking. The impaired blood supply to the brain can cause disturbances of sleep with nightmares. Another abnormality results from the limit to the volume of blood the ventricle can contain, while usual loads continue to be presented by the atrium. A limit is reached with damming back an increased load into the atrium, which also can hold only a limited amount. The left atrium continues to receive a usual load from the lungs through the pulmonary veins, some of which is dammed back into the lungs when the dilated atrium can hold no more. The damming back of blood flow engorges the lungs resulting in excess seepage of water in the blood through the capillary walls and the lining of the normally dry air spaces. The excess water displaces air in the lungs and reduces the transport of oxygen into capillaries. Small specialized organs of the nervous system detect the decrease in oxygen in circulating blood. These organs respond by sending nerve impulses to the central nervous system to increase the rate of breathing, which is involuntary. This causes patients to complain of difficulty in breathing, which is a common symptom of heart failure.

The backing up of blood flow can be transmitted to all organs with abnormalities of the liver, gastrointestinal system and kidneys. Water also seeps out through capillaries in the legs, which causes swelling of the legs below the knees. Swollen ankles are characteristic of heart failure but also occur for other reasons.

Treatment of Heart Failure

The good news is that there are very effective ways of treating heart failure. Mechanical problems such as obstructed valves can be corrected surgically with artificial valves. The ultimate surgery is a heart transplant, which is not a practical solution. Artificial hearts are being developed, which may become practical. The fact is that most causes of heart failure are effectively treated with drugs. The key drugs include digitalis and drugs called ACE-inhibitors, Beta-blockers, and aldactones. The interesting feature of all these drugs is that it is not known exactly why they are so effective. The specific chemical way they act is simply not known. A popular garden plant called foxglove (*sp. Digitalis purpurea*) was discovered over a century ago to relieve the symptoms of heart failure. Subsequent studies showed that the key ingredient in the leaf of the plant was a complex chemical called digitalis. It was the major drug among others used to treat heart failure until about twenty years ago when new drugs were developed that maintained normal blood pressures in hypertensive patients. Experience with these drugs revealed that they were remarkably effective in treating those patients who also had heart failure. Digitalis is still used but these newer drugs have led to prolonged life spans beyond the range possible with digitalis alone.

An encouraging outcome of all the continuing studies on these drugs is new information about healing in heart disease. Heart muscle is a very specialized tissue, like nerve cells, and scientists have always had the concept that such specialized tissues can't regenerate the way new skin regenerates after an abrasion. The unexpected relief of symptoms of heart failure followed by actual improvement in the heart's performance suggested that regeneration of heart muscle is possible. Investigation of this possibility has produced evidence that regeneration can occur. Evidence has even been discovered that nerve cells can also regenerate. Investigation of the mechanisms that enable regeneration assures exciting new developments in treatments.

B. The Immune System

The immune system is like the police and armed forces rolled into one, which protects us from all sorts of infectious germs and toxic foreign substances. The saliva of insect bites and poison ivy are common sources of toxins. The system consists of a large variety of different types of millions of cells that work as a team. All of them are produced in the bone marrow side by side with red cells and circulate in the bloodstream. Each has a specific action in the defense against an infectious agent or toxic substance.

The first line of defense is a cell called a polymorphnuclear leukocyte, or PMN for short. The PMNs can be compared to local police because they are constantly doing their part to destroy germs, which get a foothold in our tissues and bloodstream. We normally live at peace with all sorts of germs that infest our mouths and intestines. We even benefit from the presence of some bacteria, which produce vitamins for us. Trivial microscopic injuries constantly occur in the skin and in the lining protecting the walls of our mouths, intestines, urinary, and reproductive systems. The breaks cause microscopic hemorrhages and permit entry of germs. The PMNs in the spilled blood engulf the bacteria and destroy them. The rubble of these miniscule injuries also attracts reinforcements of PMNs for a thorough clean-up. Chewing on hard candy or brushing teeth can result in these silent injuries.

Blood consists of a large variety of millions of cells floating in a protein-rich fluid called plasma. The most common cell type is the red cell, which transports oxygen from the lungs to the tissues. Red cells make up most of the blood volume. The remaining cells include those of the immune system and most of them are them are PMNs and lymphocytes. Lymphocytes represent the armed forces of the immune system. Lymphocytes all look the same under the microscope but play many different roles like soldiers wearing identical uniforms but each specialized in some way. They also congregate in hundreds or thousands of outposts like army bases called lymph nodes throughout the body. These are discrete small oval organs varying in size from pinheads to beans and are interconnected by their own circulatory system called the lymphatic system. This is a network of thin-walled vessels that transport excess fluids absorbed from the tissues and join together to form large tubular ducts, which drain into large veins entering the heart. This tissue fluid constantly arises from the bloodstream itself, by seeping through the walls of capillaries, and maintains a watery environment for all cells.

The amazing actions of lymphocytes involve the participation of two cell types called B and T cells. Specialized cells, called antigen presenting cells or APC cells, act as agents of an intelligence system and engulf the foreign material, whether a toxin or an organism, and break it down into identifying components. The components are brought to both B and T cells and triggers each to respond in different ways. The B cells manufacture a protein called an immunoglobulin, which couples with the foreign protein and neutralizes it. The astounding fact about this ability is that for every conceivable foreign protein in the world there is a B lymphocyte among millions whose only purpose in life is to manufacture the only immunoglobulin that can neutralize it. The offending protein could be in the toxic saliva of a bee sting, or part of the wall of an infectious germ. We are born with all of these millions of diverse lookout B cells. The responding B cell transforms into a plasma cell and rapidly multiplies into millions more plasma cells.

Plasma cells have a special function. They are capable of producing a protein called an immunoglobulin, which can specifically combine with and make harmless an offending foreign substance. The substance could be on the surface of a microorganism, which enables other immune cells to feed on it. It could be a harmful substance like a snake poison, whose harmful component can be inactivated by being combined with immunoglobulin and eliminated as waste. The remarkable feature of plasma cells is that our bodies contain countless lymphocytes, each of which can transform into a specific plasma cell. Each one is capable of producing only one kind of globulin, which can only combine with the specific foreign substance it was created to neutralize. This is mind boggling because of the seeming unlimited number of possible foreign substances. The plasma cell with the appropriate globulin is stimulated to multiply rapidly as soon as the foreign substance is identified and produces sufficient globulin to neutralize the invasive dose.

The APC cells bring the same foreign marker to T cells as to the B cells. Each T cell is also endowed with the ability to respond to a specific foreign protein among millions. If the protein is a component of a virus living within infected target cells or a foreign protein on any other cell, T cells called cytotoxic or killer T cells kill the affected cells. If it is a toxin of any sort a specific T cell called a "helper" T cell responds by multiplying and "helping" the reacting B cells to multiply and transform into plasma cells to make the specific immunoglobulin.

Helper T cells also modulate the activities of killer cells and produce a variety of proteins called cytokines, which affect other complex reactions of the immune system. There are also "suppressor" T cells, which tone down the many reactions of the immune system.

The public became aware of the importance of the immune system when the global epidemic of the new virus disease called AIDS (Adult Immune Deficiency Syndrome) began in 1980. Different viruses have a predilection for different target organs, such as the skin, nervous system, and liver. The main targets of the AIDS virus are T helper lymphocytes resulting in deaths due to rampant infections. AIDS has shown that the immune system is necessary for life.

The immune system can be a double-edged sword when it attacks proteins of cells of normal organs. Like border guards checking identification papers, there are safeguards for the immune system to recognize normal tissues. The failure of these safeguards results in many diseases, which are called the "autoimmune diseases." Examples are rheumatoid arthritis, rheumatic fever, lupus erythematosis, and multiple sclerosis. There are no other common names for these illnesses. Intensive research is devoted to understanding exactly what disables the immune system from recognizing normal tissues.

C. Studies on Diagnostic Errors

An early study of the frequency of diagnostic errors disclosed at autopsy was done at the Case Western Reserve University Hospital in 1919 (1). The result was an error rate of 60%, which reflected the degree of uncertainties of medical practice at that time. One must understand that this error rate was not a measure of all medical practice, but only of a population of patients who had a lethal disease and died. The error rate of all medical practice has always been unknowable.

The most recent review of all similar surveys was published in 2003 (2) by investigators at the University of California, Baylor University, and Stanford University. This was a comprehensive review of 53 postmortem studies, which were done from 1966 to 2002. The numbers of autopsies reported from each hospital ranged from 41 to 2,067 cases and totaled 8,981. The results focused on the answers to two questions: what was the percentage of missed diagnoses involving the primary cause of death, called major errors, and what was the percentage of missed diagnoses in patients who might have benefited if the correct diagnoses had been made, called Class I errors. It became clear from repeated prior studies from individual institutions that the majority of misdiagnosed patients would not have benefited if the correct diagnoses were known. For example, a patient with terminal cancer would not have benefited if a missed terminal heart attack had been diagnosed before death. The results indicated that "...a contemporary U.S. institution...could observe a major error rate from 8.4% to 24.4% and a Class I error rate of 4.1% to 6.7%."

One of the investigators who had published a well-known study in 1983 (3) made an insightful comment on his similar results: "Our missed diagnoses did not represent malpractice or negligence but rather indicated that advances in medicine have left a residuum of obscure diagnoses, thus preserving the value of the autopsy." The reasons for the "residuum of obscure diagnoses" were made clear in a study published in 1989 (4) based on a little-known rigorous analysis of medical fallibility published in 1976 (5). Briefly, the reasons are vast voids in medical knowledge and Nature's role in producing unique misleading expressions of diseases.

D. Two Common Diagnostic Errors

Two of the more common diagnoses found postmortem in cases with mistaken diagnoses illustrate the basic reasons for inevitable medical fallibility. One is death in the elderly due to silent infections without warning symptoms. These infections often occur in patients being treated for other major diseases, with symptoms that mask the signs of any new major problem like a fatal infection. It is also known that symptoms and signs such as pain and fever that alert physicians may be blunted in the elderly and easily missed. This problem illustrates Nature's role in varying disease behavior to misleading extremes and also our voids in knowledge. A laboratory test that can reveal silent infections is feasible but dependent on insufficient knowledge about natural chemical reactions to infection. This new information could lead to laboratory tests to screen patients for serious silent infections.

Another common example is unexpected fatal pulmonary embolism, which is the obstruction of all the blood flow in the main arteries to the lungs by large jammed blood clots. This is a diagnostic problem of all adults, young and old due primarily to insufficient knowledge about blood clotting. This now makes it impossible to develop screening tests, which would reveal those individuals prone to overactive clotting.

They might benefit from lifelong blood thinning or other treatments. Pulmonary emboli can also cause misleading presenting symptoms. For example, the first few blood clots that enter the arteries of the lungs may cause a type of chest pain and other symptoms that are typically seen in heart attacks due to coronary arteriosclerosis.

E. A Comparison of Traditional and New Technological Diagnostic Methods

The explosion of extraordinary technologies has improved diagnostic accuracy, but has not eliminated uncertainty in medical practice. Doctors dread the anxiety of uncertainty and keenly apply the new technologies seeking freedom from fear. Their exuberance has led many of them to presume that faultless practice is not only possible but also the expected standard. Many doctors actually consider the autopsy obsolete. This disabling delusion roused two investigators to measure the real weight of the new technologies in diagnostic accuracy. These two well-known studies were among those included in the comprehensive review cited above (3, 6).

The postmortem diagnoses served as scientific controls on diagnoses based only on the new methods. The results of diagnoses based on new technologies were assigned to one of three categories, namely, conclusive, misleading, or inconclusive. The combined results of both reviews were 21.5% conclusive, 6.0% misleading and 72.5% inconclusive.

Again, these results apply only to autopsied cases. The value of these procedures in the living has not been as reliably studied, but there is no question that they have improved diagnostic accuracy.

One of the two studies (6) also included the weights of the two basic procedures in clinical diagnosis—the clinical history and the physical examination. These are the first tools used to make diagnoses and are still standard procedure. The clinical history is the story of the patient's illness obtained from the patient in response to questioning by the doctor. The physical examination is familiar to all. The results were that the history provided conclusive information in 73% of cases. The physical examination scored 62%. These are impressive scores as compared to the new technologies. The data illustrate why these subjects are of such fundamental importance for medical students to learn and for practicing doctors to apply. The concern is that busy doctors cannot devote the necessary time to the history and physical examination and depend too heavily on the new technologies.

References

1. Karsner, HT, Rothschild, L, Crump, ES. (1919) "Clinical diagnoses as Compared with Autopsy Findings in Six Hundred Cases." *Journal of the American Medical Association* 73:666-669.

2. Shojania, KG, Burton, EC, McDonald, KM, Goldman, L. (2003) "Changes in Rates of Autopsy-Detected Diagnostic Errors over Time." *Journal of the American Medical Association* 289: 2849-2856.

3. Goldman, L, Sayson, R, Robbins, S, Cohn, LH, Bettmann, M, Weisberg, M. (1983) "The Value of the Autopsy in Three Medical Eras." *The New England Journal of Medicine* 308:1000-1005.

4. Anderson, RE, Hill, RB, Key, CR. (1989) "The Sensitivity and Specificity of Clinical Diagnostics During Five Decades. Toward an Understanding of Necessary Fallibility." *Journal of the American Medical Association* 261: 1610-1617.

5. Gorovitz, S, MacIntyre, A. (1976) "Toward a Theory of Medical Fallibility." *Journal of Medicine and Philosophy* 1:51-71.

6. Kirsch, W, Schafii, C. (1996) "Misdiagnoses at a University Hospital in Four Medical Eras." *Medicine* 75:29-40.

Acknowledgments

I am deeply grateful to my physician, Dr. Michael Grey, who motivated me to write this book. He helped me realize that such a memoir might be an effective way of introducing to the public the idea that infallible medical practice is not possible. My good fortune continued when I met two encouraging friends. One is Razi Sharafieh, a video production specialist, who extended his hand to help me and became my co-author. Razi has a keen interest in medicine as well as a gifted sense of public relations, which was indispensable to a more reader-friendly organization of the contents and explanation of technical material. He also initiated all of the illustrations and wrote the conclusion, which is the highlight of the book. I am also grateful to Razi's daughter, Roshanak, a geneticist, who provided constructive criticism by reviewing the book, which led to important changes and additions. Razi's wife, Soghra, provided us with happy memories of working and eating together as a family in a joyous atmosphere of creativity. I am deeply grateful to her. Another friend is Justin Stafford, a physicist and mathematician, who is deeply interested in medicine, and experienced as a writer and medical reporter. He introduced me to the finer points of writing style with key references, which made me wonder how I ever wrote anything without this knowledge. He has also been a great counselor. Dr. Ellen Eisenberg, an oral pathologist, was another great counselor, who helped me present some controversial ideas in the least pejorative way possible. I emphasize that I am solely responsible for everything printed in this book. I am deeply grateful to my own family including my wife, Margo, and two sons, Kenneth and Perry, for their support, criticisms, and patience.

Index

A

abdomen, 58–59
ACE-inhibitors, 19, 62, 109–110, 131
Ackerman, Lauren V., 45, 48–49
Addison's disease, 94–96
adrenal glands, 94–95
AIDS (Adult Immune Deficiency Syndrome), 104–105, 134
aldactones, 19, 131
Alzheimer's disease, 74, 79
amino acids, 77, 78
ampulla, 51, 52, 53–54, 57
amyloid, 22
amyloidosis, 22
angina pectoris, 83, 98
angiography, 61–62
anti-coagulant therapy, 95–96
antigen presenting cells (APC), 133
aorta, 84, 85, 129
aortic valve, 129, 130
APC cells, 133
Armed Forces Institute of Pathology (AFIP), 45
arteries
    blood flow through, 127, 128
    calibers of, 97
    contraction and dilatation of, 61, 97, 98–99
    occlusion of, 58
    polyarteritis nodosa in, 85
    versus veins, 125–126

arteriosclerosis
    coronary, 83
    effects of, 58, 86
    and heart block, 89
    symptoms of, 98
artificial hearts, 131
artificial kidneys, 13
artificial valves, 131
aspiration pneumonia, 74
Atlas of Tumors of the Breast, 64
atraumatic fat embolization, 117–120
atrioventricular node, 88, 89
atriums, 127, 128–129, 130
Auerbach, Oscar, 38–39
autoimmune diseases, 134
autopsies
    of abdomen, 58–59
    and applied scientists, 6
    and diagnosis reconsiderations, 23–24
    and diagnostic accuracy, 137
    importance of, 135
    infections due to, 104–105
    of intestines, 59
    for nervous system degeneration, 74–75
    and organ diseases, 3
    origins of, 3
    for source of heart failure, 83–86

B

bacterial endocarditis, 84
bactrim, 104
barium enemas, 47
B cells, 133
Bedford Sanitarium, 20
bends, 116
benign parathyroid tumor, 23
benign tumors, 23, 32–33
Beta-blockers, 19, 62, 109–110, 131
bile ducts, 50, 51, 52
biopsies, 110
Block, Robert, 21
blood
    circulation of, 125–129, 130
    fat levels in, 119
    plasma of, 132
    thinning, 93, 136
blood clots
    anti-coagulant therapy for, 95–96
    by bacterial endocarditis, 84
    symptoms of, 93
    treating, 93
    in veins, 93
blood flow, 125–129, 130
blood loss, 58
blood plasma, 116–117
blood pressure, 17–18
blood stem cell transplant, 113–114
blood thinner, 93, 136
body temperature, 125
bone tumors, 43–45
brain, 73–74
breast cancer, 63–64, 69–71
breathing problems
    causes of, 93, 103
    and heart failure, 130
    postpartum, 109–110
bronchopneumonia, 87
Buchberg, Abraham, 21

C

cancer
    in aortic wall, 85
    breast, 63–65, 69–71
    cervical, 56
    clear cell carcinoma, 38, 39
    colon, 35–36
    defense against, 39–40
    in femur, 43–45
    and frozen sections, 46–47
    giant cell carcinoma of the thyroid gland, 85
    growth of, 34–36
    and immune system, 39–40
    of kidneys, 37–38, 39
    liposarcoma, 30
    lung, 34–35, 37, 87
    lymphoma, 89, 103, 104, 116
    metastatic, 37–38, 87, 88, 93–94
    misdiagnosis of, 100–102
    multiple myeloma, 23–25
    pancreatic (*see* pancreatic cancer)
    small cell, 34–35
    spontaneous regression of, 37–40
    and tuberculosis, 34
    tumors (*see* tumors)
    and weight loss, 16
    and X-rays, 16–17
cancer growth, 34–36
capillaries, 117, 127, 129
cardiac catheterization, 19
cardiomyopathy, 18–19, 110
cartilaginous tumor, 44
CAT scan, 40, 96

cerebral cortex, 73–74
cerebral edema, 87
cerebral swelling, 86
cervical cancer, 56
chest wall tumor, 29
chylomicrons, 119–120
circulation time, 17–18, 19
circulatory system, 125–129
clinical history, 137
clinico-pathologic conference, 5
collagen, 112–113
colon cancer, 35–36
colonoscope, 47
comas, 74
conduction system, 88
contaminated needles, 105
Coons, H., 35
cornea, 75
coronary angiogram, 98
coronary arteriosclerosis, 83
coronary artery disease, 83, 98
cortisone, 94–95
Creutzfeld-Jakob disease (CJD), 74–79
cytokines, 134
cytotoxic T cells, 133

D

death, common cause of, 58
dementia, 73–74
diagnoses
    of Addison's disease, 93–96
    of blood clots, 93
    of breast cancer, 69–71
    of cardiomyopathy, 110
    in clinico-pathologic conference, 5
    of Creutzfeld-Jakob disease (CJD), 73–75
    of heart disease, 17–19
    of heart failure, 32–33
    of intestinal polyps, 47–49
    of lymphoma, 66–68, 103
    of metastatic cancer, 37–38
    methods for, 137–138
    of multiple myeloma, 23–24
    of pancreatic cancer, 53–55, 57
    postmortem (*see* autopsies)
    proven versus disease of unknown cause, 6
    review of, 46–47
    unpredictability in, 37–39
    and weight loss, 16
    and X-rays, 16
diagnostic angiography, 61–62
diagnostic errors, 135–136. *See also* misdiagnoses
diagnostic methods, 137–138
diffuse hyperplasia, 24
digitalis treatment, 18, 61, 131
diseases
    Addison's disease, 94–96
    Alzheimer's, 74, 79
    arteriosclerosis, 58
    autoimmune, 134
    cancer (*see* cancer)
    chronic, 13
    coronary artery disease, 83
    Creutzfeld-Jakob disease (CJD), 74–79
    deadly, 13
    discovery of, 58–62
    endometriosis, 48
    fat embolization, 117–120
    heart (*see* heart disease; heart failure)
    hyperparathyroidism, 23–25
    infectious (*see* infections)

jaundice, 63, 65
of kidney, 13–14
leprosy, 14–15
low flow syndrome, 58–65
mad cow disease, 77
pancreatitis, 59
Parkinson's, 79
pernicious anemia, 114
Pneumocystis carinii pneumonia (PCP), 103–105
pneumonia, 74
polyarteritis nodosa, 59–60, 84–85
primary pulmonary hypertension, 97
progressive dementia, 74
rheumatic fever, 32, 129–130
scleroderma, 112
systemic sclerosis, 112–114
tuberculosis, 20–22, 34
DNA (deoxyribonucleic acid), 77, 78
Dockerty, Malcolm, 55–57
doubling time, 35–36
dwarfism, 76–77

E

edema, 93
Eisenberg, Ellen, 141
electroencephalogram, 98
embolism, 136
endocarditis, 84
endometriosis, 48
eosinophile, 95
epilepsy, 76

F

fainting, 97–99
fatal pulmonary embolism, 136
fat embolization, 117–120
fibroadenoma, 70, 71
fibroblasts, 112–113
foxglove, 131
frozen sections
limitations of, 46–47
at Mayo Clinic, 55, 56
of pancreatic tumor, 53–55

G

Gajdusek, D. Carleton, 75
giant cell carcinoma of the thyroid gland, 85
glands
adrenal, 94–95
colon, 48
in pancreas, 51
parathyroid, 23, 24
pituitary, 76
thyroid, 85
glucose, 125
goof conferences, 46–47
Gorovitz, Samuel, 101–102
gray matter, 73–74
Grey, Michael, 141
growth hormones, 76–77

H

heart
anatomy of, 127–129
aortic valve of, 129, 130
artificial, 131
and circulatory system, 125–129
conduction system of, 88
mitral valve of, 111
nervous system of, 88
regenerating muscle in, 131
residual blood in, 129
valves of, 32, 111, 129, 130
heart attacks, 58

heart block, 88–89
heart disease
    arteriosclerosis, 89
    bacterial endocarditis, 84
    cardiomyopathy, 18–19
    coronary artery disease, 83, 98–99
    rheumatic, 111
heart failure
    cardiomyopathy, 110
    cause of, 129
    digitalis treatment for, 18, 61
    peripartum cardiomyopathy, 109–111
    progressive, 32
    and rheumatic fever, 129–130
    symptoms of, 17, 130–131
    testing for, 17–18
    treatment of, 18, 19, 61, 62, 109, 131
    undiagnosed, 114–115
heart surgery, 33
heart transplants, 131
heart tumors, 33
helper T cell, 133–134
hemoglobin, 114
Hill, Rolla B., 101–102
HIV (Human Immunodeficiency Disease Virus), 104–105
hyperparathyroidism, 23–25
hypertension, 110
hypothalamus, 96

I

immune system
    defense of cancer, 39–40
    overview of, 132–134
    and systemic sclerosis, 113
immunoglobulin, 133
infarcts, 58, 59, 60–61
infections
    amyloidosis, 22
    bacterial endocarditis, 84
    causing death, 136
    and contaminated needles, 105
    Creutzfeld-Jakob disease (CJD), 74–79
    due to autopsies, 104–105
    and lymph nodes, 66
    preventing acquisition of, 20–22
    tuberculosis, 20–22, 34
insulin, 51
insurance, xi. *See also* liability insurance
intestinal polyps, 47–49
intestines, 59, 60–61

J

Jaffee, Henry, 44
jaundice, 63, 65
Jewish Hospital of St. Louis, 39, 43–79

K

keloids, 13–14
kidney cancer, 37–38, 39
kidney disease, 13–14
killer T cells, 133
kuru, 75

L

left atrium, 33
Leiter, Louis, 13
leprosy, 14–15
liability insurance, 122
life expectancy, xi
lipoma, 69
lipoproteins, 119

liposarcoma, 30
litigation. *See* medical litigation
liver, 51, 59
low flow syndrome, 58–65
lung cancer
    metastatic, 37, 87
    small cell cancer, 34–35
lungs, 97
lymphatic system, 132–133
lymph nodes
    abnormal colon glands in, 48
    cancer in (*see* lymphoma)
    enlarged, 66
    functions of, 66, 132
lymphocytes, 132
lymphoma, 66–68, 103, 104, 116

M

mad cow disease, 77
Martinus, Willem Beijerinck, 78
Mayo Clinic, 55–57
McIntyre, Alasdair, 101–102
medical care
    expectations for, xi
    at Mayo Clinic, 55–57
medical costs, xi
medical education, 5, 6–7
medical errors, xii. *See also* misdiagnoses
medical litigation
    beginnings of, 6
    causes of, xi
    effect on medical practice, xi, 7
    ending, 121–122
    and medical costs, xi
medical practice
    dangers of, 21
    difficulties in, 6–8
    and end of litigation, 121–122

expectations for, 6–7
fallibility of, 7–8, 121
and infection, 20–22
uncertainty in, 121, 137
medical school, xii, 5, 6–7
metastatic cancer
    finding, 88
    from lungs, 87
    in lungs, 37–38
    misdiagnosis of, 93–94
Methodist Hospital, 55, 56
microscopes, 4
misdiagnoses
    of breast cancer, 63–65
    of cancer, 100–102
    Class I errors, 135
    common instances of, 136
    due to unexpected changes, 37–39
    frequency of, 135
    of heart diseases, 97–99
    of heart failure, 32–33
    major errors, 135
    of metastatic cancer, 94
mitral stenosis, 111
mitral valve, 32, 111, 129, 130
Montefiore Hospital, xii
    Bedford Sanitarium, 20
    internship at, 13–25
    pathology at, 83–89
    pathology training at, 29–40
    reputation of, 13
Morgagni, Giovanni, 3
Mount Sinai Hospital, 93–105
MRI, 40, 96
multiple myeloma, 23–24
myeloma, 23
myxoma, 33

N

National Pituitary Foundation, 76
natural healing, 37
needle aspiration biopsy, 100
nervous system, 74–79
neurologists, 98
nucleic acids, 77

O

oil red O, 117
organs
    and microscopes, 4
    recognizing disease in, 3
    See also individual organ names
orthopedists, 44–45
oxygen, 125–129

P

pancreas
    ampulla of, 51, 52, 53–54, 57
    anatomy of, 50–51, 89
pancreatic cancer
    and fat embolization, 118
    and heart block, 88–89
    nontreatment of, 51
    Whipple operation for, 50–55, 57
pancreatitis, 59
parathyroid glands, 23, 24
Parkinson's disease, 79
pathologists
    abilities of, 43
    influential, 3–4
    job of, 3–4
    risk of infection for, 104–105
    versus surgeons, 43
    tumor analysis by, 43–44

pathology
    dealing with unusual diseases in, 109–110
    defined, 3
    at Jewish Hospital of St. Louis, 43–79
    at Mayo Clinic, 55–57
    at Montefiore Hospital, 13–25, 29–40, 83–89
    at Mount Sinai Hospital, 93–105
    and new diseases, 58–62
    origins of, 3
    and polyps, 47–49
    risk of infection in, 104–105
    surgical, 4
    training in, 29–40
    uncertainty in, 121
    at University of Connecticut Health Center, 109–120
peripartum cardiomyopathy, 109–111
pernicious anemia, 114
physical examinations, 137
pituitary gland, 76
pituitary growth hormones, 76
plasma, 116–117, 132
plasma cells, 133
Pneumocystis carinii pneumonia (PCP), 103–105
pneumonia, 87
    aspiration, 74
    Pneumocystis carinii, 103–105
polyarteritis nodosa, 59–60, 84–85
polymorphnuclear leukocyte (PMN), 132
polyps, 47–49
postmortem diagnosis. *See* autopsies
potassium concentration, 94–95

pregnancy, peripartum cardiomyopathy, 109–111
primary pulmonary hypertension, 97–99
prion, 78–79
progressive dementia, 73–74
progressive heart failure, 32
protein infectious agent, 78–79
proteins, 77, 78
Prusiner, Stanley B., 77–78, 79
pulmonary embolism, 136

R

red blood cells, 127, 132
residual blood, 129
residual tumors, 30–31
rheumatic fever, 32, 111, 129–130
rheumatic heart disease, 111
Rokitansky, Carl, 3

S

Saint Mary's Hospital, 56
scleroderma, 112
sclerosing adenosis, 71
Sharafieh, Razi, 141
sigmoidoscope, 47
sinoatrial nodes, 88, 89
skin grafts, 30
small cell cancer, 34–35
small intestines, 51–53
Social Security Act, xi
soft tissue tumors, 29–31
spontaneous regression, 37–40
Stafford, Justin, 141
Stanley, Wendell M., 78
stem cell transplant, 113–114
stenosis, 32
Stewart, Fred, 64, 71
stomach, 59
Stout, Arthur Purdy, 38, 39, 45, 46
strokes, 58, 86
suppressor T cells, 134
surgeons, 43
surgery
    on heart, 33
    for small cell cancer, 34–36
    for tuberculosis, 34
    tumor excisions, 29–31
surgical pathology, 4, 46–47
swelling, 130
systemic sclerosis, 112–114

T

T cells, 133–134
thyroid gland, 85
Tsai, Conrad, 84
tuberculosis
    and cancer, 34
    patients of, 21–22
    preventing acquisition of, 20–22
    treatment of, 20–22, 34
    undetected cases of, 22
tumors
    of ampulla, 57
    analysis of, 43–44
    bone, 43–45
    in breasts, 69–71
    cartilaginous, 44
    in chest wall, 29–31
    excision of, 29–31
    fibroadenoma, 70, 71
    in heart, 33
    lipoma, 69
    liposarcoma, 30
    malignant versus benign, 43–45
    myxomas, 33

pancreatic, 53–55
parathyroid, 23
recurrent, 44–45
residual, 30–31
sclerosing adenosis, 71
in soft tissues, 29–31
in thyroid gland, 85
undifferentiated malignant, 85
uterine, 63, 65

U

ultrasounds, 33
undifferentiated malignant tumor, 85
University of Connecticut Health Center, xi-xii, 109–120
uterine tumors, 63, 65

V

veins, 125–126, 128–129
ventricles, 127, 128–129, 130
ventricular fibrillation, 83
ventricular tachycardia, 99
Virchow, Rudolf, 4
vision loss, 73–74
vitamin B-12 deficiency, 114

W

weight loss, 16, 96
Welch, William, 4
Whipple operation, 50–55, 57
white blood cells, 95

X

X-rays
of abdomen, 58–59
and metastatic cancer, 88
and tuberculosis, 34
use of, 16–17

Z

Zimmerman, Harry M., 30, 38, 103–104, 118–119

978-0-595-34569-4
0-595-34569-7

Printed in the United States
43468LVS00004B/511-516